8 Weeks to
Vibrant
Health

8 Weeks to
Vibrant Health

**A Take-Charge Plan for Women
to Correct Imbalances, Reclaim Energy
and Restore Well-being**

HYLA CASS, M.D.
& KATHLEEN BARNES

Take
Charge
BOOKS

Brevard,
North Carolina

Take Charge Books
Brevard, NC 28712
www.takechagebooks.com

Library of Congress Cataloging-in-Publication Data

LCCN: 2008923708
ISBN: 978-0-9815818-0-4

This book was originally published in 2005 by McGraw-Hill, New York, NY.

Editor: Kathleen Barnes
Typesetting/Graphic design: Gary A. Rosenberg
Cover design: Jim English

Printed in the United States of America

10   9   8   7   6   5   4   3   2   1

CONTENTS

ACKNOWLEDGMENTS

My first appreciation is for my parents, who have unfailingly supported and encouraged me. My late father Dr. Isadore Cass, a physician and scholar, was my great teacher and role model, and my mother Miriam Cass continues to be my best cheerleader. Alison Schur, my daughter and best production yet, her wonderful husband Seth, and their precious son, Jacob, make it all worth it. My co-author and friend, Kathleen has been a joy to work with — smart, resourceful, warm, humorous, and a true kindred spirit. Special thanks to my friend and exceptional author Mary Shomon, who came up with the original book idea. My dear friend and fine health writer Nan Fuchs PhD gave me great advice and encouragement, and helped to make this a better book. And much appreciation goes to my many friends who were always there when I needed them, including Toni Galardi, Debra Bass, Debbie Friedman, Ruth Ziemba, my sisters Sharon, Judy and Elaine and their husbands. I also want to thank my dear colleagues who were always available to answer questions and give me feedback: Drs. Cynthia Watson, Murray Susser, David Katzin, Jacob Teitelbaum, Michael Rosenbaum, Shari Lieberman, and Ann Louise Gittleman, among others. My biggest thanks goes to my patients and readers who teach me new things every day, and inspire me to do and be my best.

—Hyla Cass, MD

To Hyla, my deepest respect. In working with her, I found the spirit of true sisterhood. What began as a professional relationship blossomed into a deep friendship that we both will treasure for years to come. I am deeply appreciative of the advice and encouragement of my many friends at the American Society of Journalists who haveopened whole new vistas for me in the realm of publishing. Thanks are also in order for my friends Sabra Hammond, Diane Hamilton and Libby Mojica and my sister, Julie Barnes, for their sage advice, strong shoulders and willing ears. Most of all, my deepest love and thanks to Joe Castro, my husband, life mate, and best friend, for his unfailing love, support, and smoothies.

—Kathleen Barnes

PREFACE

Kathleen and I have made every effort to make this book complete and accurate. However, because it's not about the conventional or the tried-and-true, there are varying opinions and schools of thought, and even conflicting research (as in much of medicine) on many of the topics covered here. Also, due to constantly changing information, limits in both time and space, and our being human, there will invariably be some errors and omissions.

Fortunately I have a website (www.drcass.com) which is constantly being updated with the newest information. In fact, I see this book as the initial step in an evolving process, and I invite you to participate online. Please e-mail me not only your comments, criticisms, questions, and additions, but also share your own health makeover experiences. I'd like the website to be a place for active exchange, where all of us can learn from each other.

Gone are the days when a doctor—or a book—could claim to have all the answers! In my clinical practice, I invite my patients to enter into more of a partnership relationship, where we work together to solve problems and optimize their health. With this book and my website, I invite readers also to become partners in an ongoing journey of well-being that I hope will last long after the last page has been read.

—Hyla Cass, MD

INTRODUCTION

There are almost 109 million women over the age of 18 in the United States. Because of our fast-paced lifestyle; the accelerating pressure of career, family, and relationships; and the shift toward more equality in our social structure, we develop more health concerns by the day. We are also more susceptible than men to many conditions, including depression, chronic fatigue syndrome, weight gain, and, of course, hormonal swings. I hear the same laments over and over from young women, middle-aged women, and older women, whether in my office, by e-mail, at public appearances, or even at social gatherings:

"I'm always tired—it doesn't matter how long I sleep!"

"I can't catch up on everything I need to do."

"What can I do about my weight problems? I'm disgusted with myself!"

"I'm always feeling down in the dumps."

"My whole body hurts! If it's not my back, it's my shoulders or my feet."

"My PMS is actually getting worse as I get older!"

"I have absolutely no sex drive!"

"I had no idea menopause would be this bad. Between the hot flashes and night sweats, I'm miserable!"

"I'm totally confused about hormone replacement therapy. My doctor says there is no other choice—either take HRT with its risks, or suffer!"

And, from most of these women I hear, "My doctor says they are just signs of normal aging or that I'm just stressed and depressed—meaning that it's really all in my head!"

Nonetheless, problems with fatigue, sleep, anxiety, depression, weight, pain, hormones, and memory are real and often debilitating. Part of the problem is that most doctors simply don't have time to delve into the reasons for these symptoms. They may have only 10 minutes to hear out a patient, make a diagnosis, and then prescribe a pain medication, a diet pill, an antidepressant, or a sleeping pill.

If you have felt frustrated at not being truly heard and discouraged that everything you've done to try solve your health problems has failed, take heart. You're not alone, and you're not without tools to become your own health detective.

I have devised the Vibrant Health Plan based on my decades of experience in treating hundreds of women of all ages. As a conventionally trained physician with a specialty in psychiatry, I have incorporated nutrition and other natural techniques into my practice for more than 20 years.

At the core of this practice is a set of beliefs that have served my patients well:

- Treat the whole person—mind, body, spirit, and environment.

- Look for the deepest root problems beneath the symptoms, which includes using the best that science has to offer.

- Apply a continuum of treatments, always beginning with the safest, most natural, and most benign.

CRUSADE FOR REFORM

I am often asked how I became such a crusader for the reform of conventional medicine. The fact is, there was no single turning point or moment of enlightenment. It has been a long process, beginning with my earliest family life.

My father was a general practitioner who practiced out of our home in Toronto, Canada. From an early age, I recall following him around on his medical rounds at the hospital and going along on house calls. A caring and conscientious GP in an old-fashioned practice, I saw him practice integrated medicine long before that term was coined. Available and responsive, he ministered to his patients with care and skill. He would talk to me about what he was doing, assuming I understood, never talking down to me. Looking back now, I realize that as the doctor's apprentice, I learned a great deal about the spirit and art of medicine, and even about practical aspects of diagnosis and treatment.

Moving forward many years, I studied medicine at the University of Toronto School of Medicine and then interned at the Los Angeles County–USC School of Medicine. I was struck by the serious class divisions in the system of medical care, experiencing culture shock as I was exposed for the first time to a clearly segregated medical care system with serious divisions based on socioeconomic status. In Canada, health coverage is universal, and I had not seen such a disparity in terms of quality of care and the respect given to patients and their families. Both my experience with my father and my medical school training had already given me a more humane and holistic view of medical care, in contrast to the prevailing mechanized, impersonal system.

My interest in a more relational, holistic approach, coupled with an appreciation for the mind-body connection, led me to psychiatry. During my residency at Cedars-Sinai/UCLA Medical Center, I eventually found that the standard "couch and Prozac" combination of psychoanalytic and pharmacological treatments had their limitations.

I was drawn to a more personal approach to patients, where therapists were more directly caring and interactive with their patients. I discovered art therapy with Helen Landgarten, then guided imagery and other more cutting-edge interactive techniques such as Voice Dialogue with Hal Stone. Not only did these methods work more quickly, but they clearly could affect the body in many ways, from relieving more obvious symptoms to boosting the immune system.

Then, during my family therapy fellowship, I discovered the "systems approach," where the "identified patient" was not necessarily the true problem! It wasn't just Johnny who was the "bad kid" or Jenna who was the depressed adolescent. In fact, there were secret family issues (Mom's depression, Dad's gambling) that had unbalanced the whole family dynamic, and the *children's problems* were the *family's symptoms.* Treatment would be successful only so far as the underlying issues (i.e., the parents' problems) were uncovered and healed.

By the same token, I became aware that the symptoms my patients reported were just messages that something in their body systems was awry. They were clues that needed closer evaluation in order to uncover the real cause. I paid more attention to the mind-body connection and the doctor-patient relationship.

I carried what I had learned into my new medical practice and began to explore the influences of nutrition and lifestyle on health. I observed how imbalance in the body can affect the mind. The brain, after all, is an organ, affected by its internal physiological environment.

It became obvious to me that psychotherapy is more effective once the brain is functioning properly. I went on to discover how many typical psychiatric complaints—anxiety, depression, PMS, even schizophrenia—are frequently related to biochemical imbalances. These can range from low blood sugar, viral and fungal infections, hormonal imbalances, allergies, and toxic overload to deficiencies of specific nutrients.

I am able to diagnose these conditions with the appropriate laboratory tests that give a scientific basis for treatment decisions. Then I can often help correct the imbalances with natural approaches, including the use of well-researched nutritional supplements. In contrast, conventional physicians are most likely to prescribe first and test second, if at all, with problematic results.

THE THIRD LEADING CAUSE OF DEATH

Studies show that doctors are the third leading cause of death, accounting for 250,000 deaths per year. They don't do it intentionally, but due to a lack of knowledge, errors, and excessive influence from drug companies, that is the end result.

There is little to counterbalance the over-prescribing of drugs, despite the fact that according to one study, there are more than 100,000 deaths per year in hospitals alone, due to medications taken as prescribed. That's not taking into account drugs that were improperly prescribed or medication-related disability that, while not fatal, takes a huge toll. Or the deaths that were attributed to the condition but were really due to the treatment.

In my move toward "integral" or holistic psychiatry, I found myself treating a variety of medical conditions, from chronic fatigue to irritable bowel syndrome. Patients don't walk into our offices as disembodied heads. Our bodies do not separate into specialized compartments for the convenience of cardiologists, allergists, endocrinologists, or gastroenterologists. You can't get to the right diagnosis and treatment without looking at all systems!

Every symptom reflects an imbalance somewhere in the body's systems. Conventional medicine has segmented the body into the various specialties, and often fails to address the reality of interactive systems.

Holistic or *integrative* medicine, on the other hand, addresses the interactive systems of the whole person. The patient is evaluated in a variety of ways and supplied with specific health prescriptions—for supplements, foods, exercise, natural hormones, mind-body techniques, and even prescription drugs when indicated. Moreover, the individual has to partner with the doctor in this process, both to carry out the regimen and to give feedback in order to fine-tune the program.

Compared to drug therapy, natural treatments offer safer, more user-friendly solutions with far fewer and less harmful side effects. They work with the body's chemistry rather than adding what can be toxic substances to an already impaired body.

A CASE IN POINT

I remember one early patient in particular, a 55-year-old college teacher named Jean whose story is pretty typical. She was being treated by her internist for high blood pressure, osteoporosis, and heart palpitations. She was referred to me, a psychiatrist, because of her anxiety, depression, and insomnia. I could find no obvious psychological explanation for these symptoms, except maybe for the stress of her physical illness. She was taking an array of medications, with their attendant side effects. Based on some simple lab tests and my own clinical experience, I determined that a likely common cause was a magnesium deficiency.

After a brief trial on this inexpensive and common mineral, together with a multivitamin-mineral formula and essential fatty acids, Jean was able to decrease her medications. Encouraged by this result, she trusted me enough to eliminate some foods to which she was allergic, which helped her even more. In a short time, not only were her anxiety, depression, and insomnia gone, but she soon was medication-free, depending instead on a list of supplements (I added a few to those mentioned here) to restore her normal body chemistry.

As an integrative physician, I see cases like Jean's all day long, with sometimes seemingly simple solutions to what appear to be complex conditions. Part of the problem may even stem from the prescribed medications.

Situations like Jean's leave me with the following questions:

1. Why had Jean's internist been unaware of her mineral deficiency, or even, of its possibility? Why didn't he at least give her a basic multivitamin-mineral formula?

2. Why give prescription drugs first? This approach is like unplugging the noisy smoke alarm instead of looking for the fire!

And, more pointedly, why is the prevailing standard of medical practice so *symptom- and drug-oriented,* especially when this approach so clearly fails to serve the patient?

One answer is all too clear: through sales representatives, medical journal ads, research articles, and conventions, the pharmaceutical industry is the main source of education for many physicians in practice. The bad news is that drugs are expensive and often cause more harm than they cure. For example, the nonsteroidal anti-inflammatory drugs (NSAIDs) for arthritis can cause severe gastric irritation and even ulcers. Or, as numerous human and animal studies show, the statin drugs for lowering cholesterol deplete the body of the essential nutrient coenzyme Q_{10}, which heart cells depend on for survival. This leads us to believe that statins, while certainly lowering cholesterol, may be doing more harm than good. In his 22-page, fully referenced report reviewing this issue, researcher Dr. Peter Lonsjoen recommends that all statins be labeled with a warning to take them with 100–200 mg of coenzyme Q_{10} daily. Has your doctor mentioned that to you? Have you seen it in any drug ads? This is the tip of the iceberg for the complexity of the pharmaceutical industry and our health (fda.gov/ohrms/dockets/dailys/02/May02/052902/02p-0244-cp00001-02-Exhibit_A-vol1.pdf). I cover this in *Supplement Your Prescription: What Your Doctor Doesn't Know about Nutrition.*

Most doctors have minimal exposure to more natural treatments, which they dismiss as "unscientific." In fact, the science is there, published in the very same medical journals that tout drugs. The supplements that I recommend are well backed by published research.

Fortunately, this situation is changing as more doctors are encouraged by the results they observe in their patients who are incorporating natural approaches. (Hint: if you find solutions to your problems in this book, please share them with your doctors.) Physicians and even medical schools are showing greater interest in integrative medicine, which incorporates the best of both worlds.

The medical profession aside, I believe that with all the variables affecting our health and well-being, from diet and lifestyle to toxic exposure, we each need to take greater responsibility for our own health. Rather than taking our body to the doctor as we would take our car to the mechanic, we need to become participants in a working partnership in which the physician becomes a resource.

I wrote the book *Natural Highs* as a "brain handbook" to help those outside of my own office practice to learn how to change their own brain biochemistry and to orient those who were coming to see me. Now, in *8 Weeks to Vibrant Health,* I want to reach the millions of you out there who are stuck, stymied, knowing that something is wrong, but unsure of where to look for the solution. Here is a new handbook, one for the body as well as the mind.

This book is meant to help you learn as much as you can and do as much as you know how to maintain optimum health and find a doctor who is willing to join you in the process.

ABOUT KATHLEEN BARNES

Kathleen Barnes has long personal experience with alternative and complementary therapies. She taught yoga for more than 30 years while working as a foreign correspondent on three continents. She wrote a natural health column for *Woman's World* magazine for six years until the first edition of this book launched her on a new career writing and editing natural health and sustainable living books. Writing for professionals and consumers in these and other forums has deepened her understanding of the field, including a practical knowledge of what readers need, want and are able to do.

While this book is often written from my point of view as a physician, Kathleen provided her broad knowledge and years of experience in creating the core content and organization of this book.

She is currently in the process of writing her 13th book and has recently launched her newsletter and website, *Living, Naturally* at www.kathleen barnes.com.

—————————————

With our heartfelt wishes for your success in discovering or regaining a healthy balance in body, mind, and spirit, we both offer you our knowledge and experience, as well as our compassion and our commitment to helping you find your way to vibrant health.

1

YOUR VIBRANT
HEALTH PLAN

1

WEEK 1

Beginning Your Journey to Better Health

———

You can treat the leaves or you can treat the roots.
—ANCIENT CHINESE SAYING

Consider *8 Weeks to Vibrant Health* to be an operating manual for your body and mind. It is an eight-week guided program of self-education, self-evaluation and self-care. The self-scoring questionnaires will help you pinpoint areas of imbalance in these 10 major areas:

- Diet and nutrition
- Lifestyle
- Exercise
- Brain chemistry
- Sex hormones
- Thyroid and adrenal hormones
- Blood sugar
- Digestive system including yeast
- Toxins and detoxification
- Weight control

Based on your answers, you will be able to order specific lab tests for further exploration.

The second part of the book will give you detailed information on the key areas of imbalance, suggesting further testing as needed, then giving detailed recommendations to help restore balance. These include dietary modifications, natural hormones, herbs and supplements, detoxification programs and exercises. You'll create new habits that will help you move into the future with greater resilience, energy and overall health.

Here is how best to use this book:

1. It's a good idea to read the book all the way through first, to familiarize yourself with the material, including the steps you can take to resolve your health problems.

2. Work through the chapters of the eight-week *Vibrant Health Plan* one at a time, beginning with your food-mood-supplement-activity record, journal, questionnaire and lab tests, so you have an idea of where you are and where you want to end up on your journey to good health. (The lab tests appear in the early weeks so you can get the results sooner.)

3. Start incorporating the suggested dietary and lifestyle changes. Often, this will be a huge jump-start in changing how you feel. Record these in your journal.

4. Use Part 2 to dig more deeply to better understand and treat your specific problems, one at a time.

5. When you've completed the program to address one imbalance, you can start on another. Please be kind to yourself and address only one major problem at a time.

6. Work at your own pace. The suggested eight weeks is a good average, but some women may take more time, and some may take less. It depends on your starting point and your own style.

Your investigation in the first eight chapters of this book will lead you to possible root causes of your health problems. You may appear to have more than one underlying imbalance. You won't always have to handle them one after another because, in many cases, handling one major problem will resolve others, too. For example, for many women, handling hormonal imbalances will also clear up many other problems such as anxiety, depression, overweight and insomnia.

Some of your investigations may require that you see a doctor, especially if you need prescription medications or some kinds of laboratory testing. Regardless, this book will give you enough information to become a partner with your physician, working together to bring about your return to vibrant health.

Please be realistic. If, for example, you have more than 10 or 15 pounds to lose, we won't hold out false hope. You won't lose 50 or 60 pounds in the course of an eight-week program, but you will be well on your way to achieving a healthy weight.

You'll find easy ways to make better nutritional choices, to make exercise more fun, and to better understand the healing power of herbs and supplements. Most importantly, your intuition will often know what's best for you, so we'll give you some tools to help you reconnect with your inner wisdom.

The Vibrant Health Plan calls for gradual changes, so be gentle with yourself! Part of this whole program is learning to really care about yourself, your body and your feelings.

This first week, you'll start your journal and then pay close attention to what you eat and drink. This will also give you a good idea what to add to or remove from your diet. You'll get basic information on exercise as well as the importance of quality sleep and proper breathing.

STARTING A WELLNESS JOURNAL

The word journal sounds a lot like journey. In fact, your journal will become the road map on your journey to health. Besides your own reflections, your journal needs to hold extra sheets such as the ongoing food-mood-supplement-activity record, lab test results, newspaper clippings, website printouts and any other information you collect in your exploration. Include some blank sheets for your own notes, as well. We have provided a sample food-mood-supplement-activity record that you can photocopy and use in your notebook, or you can create your own. You can also download it from the book's website www.drcass.com.

Keep your journal in a handy place. In the coming weeks, you'll refer to it over and over as you assess your symptoms and create your plan to address them.

For this entire week, and for the rest of your eight-week Vibrant Health Plan, write down everything you eat and drink—meals, snacks, juices, coffee and alcohol. Include the approximate quantities as well. Your nutritional habits will become obvious as you write them down and perhaps will prompt some immediate changes. Do you eat at least five servings of fruits and vegetables a day? If not, you'll see it easily in your journal pages.

Pay attention to your *patterns* of eating and drinking, as well. Write down why you ate or drank just then (hunger, boredom, fatigue, etc.) and how you felt afterward (energized, guilty, deserving, etc.). Use a scale from 1 to 5 showing your hunger level.

Here are some examples of questions to consider when you eat:

- How were you feeling before you ate?

- Did you feel true "gut hunger"?

- Were you eating to relieve stress or a low mood?

- Were you eating or drinking out of habit and not really because of hunger or thirst?

- Did you eat hurriedly or calmly?

- Did you eat normal portions?

- How did you feel after you ate (e.g., satisfied, healthy, guilty)?

Notice whether you are eating sugar or drinking coffee to raise your mood, energy, or concentration and then having lows an hour or two afterward when you find yourself craving a doughnut or another cup of coffee. Or notice if you reach for a glass of wine to calm yourself down when you're feeling stressed.

Your symptoms list is useful in tracking food intolerances, discussed more in Chapter 14. For example, you might notice a stomach ache or diarrhea after eating dairy products or fatigue several hours after eating corn or wheat or even some great health food. Or you might not even have a reaction till the following day. Food intolerances are tricky that way and often need careful detective work to pin them down.

Also note how much you exercise: What you do, when, and for how long. Add up the total minutes spent daily. In addition to time spent at the gym or power walking or using the treadmill in the basement, walking the dog for 15 minutes counts. So do the 10 minutes you spent vacuuming the house and the

20 minutes of weeding the garden or raking leaves. Hey, even folding laundry qualifies.

You'll also log the hours you sleep each night, meaning actual sleep time, not time spent watching TV or reading in bed.

Include a line or two each day about how you feel, your energy levels and your mood.

Looking back at these entries after just a week can be a real eye-opener. It will help you see some simple ways you can make changes that will have profound effects on your health.

For a sample journal page that you can photocopy for your Wellness Journal, turn to the following page.

You may be surprised at what you discover when you read your first week's journal.

Kate, a 35-year-old full-time accountant and mother of two teenagers is a good example. Her complaint at our first meeting was, "I just can't lose those 15 pounds and I am exhausted all the time. My family doctor just told me, 'What do you expect? Full-time job, two children, it's no wonder you're tired!' But I'm not convinced. I know there are things I should be doing to improve my health, but I'm just too tired to think about them, let alone do them."

Kate had brought her preceding week's food-mood-supplement-activity record. She realized that she was getting almost no exercise and that the majority of her diet was made up of starchy carbohydrates—bread, pasta, rice and bagels. Inspired by the possibility of really changing her life, she vowed to stop the starch overload. She planned to eat a protein-rich breakfast and bring a more balanced lunch with her to work, including cut-up vegetables for snacks. She was also going to use the stairs at work instead of the elevator to get to her fourth-floor office. These were small changes, but they were a great start and would make a big difference in her life. After her initial eight weeks, Kate was well on track. She'd lost eight pounds and her exercise program had helped substantially increase her energy.

ADD WATER

You've heard this before, and it's true: you need about 64 ounces of good, pure water a day. A more exact calculation would be half your weight in ounces. For example, if you weigh 120 pounds, you'd drink 60 oz. It replenishes the

DAILY FOOD-MOOD-SUPPLEMENT-ACTIVITY RECORD

This work sheet will help you develop a clear picture of your lifestyle: eating habits, exercise, sleep, mood and supplements. For this process to be effective, keep your journal sheet with you and fill it out promptly every time you eat or drink anything including water. For the "Hunger" column, use a scale from 0 to 5: 0 = not hungry and 5 = very hungry.

Date: _____

Exercise: What _____ When _____ How long _____

Feeling before _____

Feeling after _____

Sleep: Got up _____ a.m.   Went to bed previous night _____ p.m.   Total sleep: _____ hours

How I felt today: _____

_____

TIME	FOOD/BEVERAGE	AMOUNT	HUNGER	CIRCUMSTANCES	MOOD BEFORE	MOOD AFTER	SUPPLEMENTS/MEDICATIONS

TIME	FOOD/BEVERAGE	AMOUNT	HUNGER	CIRCUMSTANCES	MOOD BEFORE	MOOD AFTER	SUPPLEMENTS/MEDICATIONS

amount of water lost in a day through the skin (sweat) and kidneys (urine). Your urine output should be two to three liters a day, clear and light yellow, unless you are taking lots of B vitamins, which makes it bright yellow. Dehydration is more common than we think. For more information, see Dr. F. Batmanghelidj's *Water: For Health, for Healing, for Life: You're Not Sick, You're Thirsty!* (Grand Central Publishing, 2003).

Avoid tap water, which can be full of contaminants and heavy metals (see Chapter 15). Caffeinated beverages don't count in your water quota, because they actually leach minerals, taking water with them as well. However, soups counts. Juices technically can contribute to your water intake, but since fruit juices (even pure fruit juices) are so high in sugar, we don't recommend them. Eat whole fruit instead. If you do drink fruit juice, make it unsweetened, and dilute it at least by half with water.

Invest in a good water purifier and drink form that at home and take along bottles when you're at work or elsewhere. The good purifiers cost in the neighborhood of $300, but you'll get some value even form the $12 pitcher-type purifiers.

Why do we need water? Our bodies are composed of 60 to 70% water. Two-thirds of it is in the cells, where it is essential for all chemical processes. The rest is in bodily fluids such as blood and in the lymphatic system, which carry nutrients to the cells and remove the toxic by-products of metabolism from the system. What's more, studies show that water restriction actually increases fat accumulation.

Here's an easy way to count your glasses of water: Fill up a 64-ounce bottle with water and refill your cup from it throughout the day until it's gone. Drink more if you like—this is just the minimum. Water is much better absorbed when you sip it throughout the day rather than gulping down a glass or two every few hours. You can substitute non-caffeinated herb teas, as well.

MAKE TIME FOR SLEEP

Sleep gets its own section in your Week 1 Vibrant Health Plan because it is so essential to all aspects of your health.

Most adults need between seven and nine hours of sleep each night for optimum health, performance, and safety.

According to the National Sleep Foundation, "When we don't get adequate sleep, we accumulate a sleep debt that can be difficult to 'pay back' if it becomes too big. The resulting sleep deprivation has been linked to health problems such as obesity and high blood pressure, negative mood and behavior, decreased productivity and safety issues in the home, on the job, and on the road."

Yet the average American gets fewer than seven hours of sleep a night, and at least two-thirds of all Americans are sleep deprived.

Make a pledge to yourself right now: Get eight hours of sleep a night, and go to bed as early as possible. Yes, naps count, to a degree, but you can't add more than one hour of napping into your sleep total because interrupted sleep isn't as deep and rejuvenating as continuous sleep.

Practicing good sleep habits will contribute to the best possible snooze once you get in bed. This means having a comfortable and comforting bedroom and turning off the TV. Taking a warm bath, drinking a glass of warm milk, and putting on some soothing music will help you get the sleep you need. Having trouble falling or staying asleep? We address this in Chapter 9 on stress reduction.

Here is one case of insomnia that illustrates some of these points. Mira, a patient of mine, noticed in her weekly journal that she was actually not sleeping very well. She was waking up several times during the night and having trouble falling back to sleep. Mira realized that there were some ways she could improve the situation. She began by not watching television before she went to bed. She also cut out her after-dinner espresso and substituted a soothing cup of chamomile tea. The result was, she was able to fall asleep more easily. However, she still needed help staying asleep, as we'll see.

BREATHE DEEPLY

You can live for a month or more without food, four days without water, but only four minutes without air. Air is the stuff of life. In fact, some Asian cultures believe a person is predestined to take only a fixed number of breaths in a lifetime, so it is a good idea to breathe deeply and slowly to prolong your life.

Predestination notwithstanding, there's no question that breathing deeply and slowly has profound effects on your body, mind, and spirit.

Deep, slow breathing brings oxygen in exchange for carbon dioxide in individual cells, where it produces the cell's energy. When we don't get enough oxygen, we get tired, cranky, and dull because of the increase in carbon dioxide levels. That's why taking a few deep breaths help recharge your cells and can change your world from dull gray to Technicolor.

Your breathing is a reflection of your emotions. When you are anxious or afraid, your breath becomes rapid and shallow. When you are happy and content, your breath becomes slow and deep. You can also use your breath to change a negative emotional situation.

Imagine you've just had near collision in traffic. Your heart is pounding, your adrenaline pumping, and your mind racing. If you simply take 10 deep, slow breaths, these physiological symptoms related to stress will disappear. So, too, will your anxiety. We'll have more about stress later. For now, remember that your breath and your mind and body are connected.

Most of us breathe too shallowly. In fact, each lung is the size of a football, and most of us are using only one-third of that capacity. Now is the time to develop the habit of breathing more deeply, so begin by spending a few short minutes every day doing just that. You'll be ahead of the game if you stop several times during the day and take a few deep breaths. See "Deep-Breathing Exercise."

DEEP-BREATHING EXERCISE

Sit comfortably in a quiet place with your spine straight.

Relax your belly muscles.

As you inhale, let your abdomen expand. Feel your diaphragm being pulled down as your lungs fill with air from the bottom to the top.

Pause briefly when you've inhaled fully.

As you exhale, gently contract your belly and squeeze the air out from top to bottom.

Repeat at your own pace.

A good resource for learning optimum breathing techniques is Michael Grant White's website, www.breathing.com.

STRETCH YOUR MUSCLES

Most of us spend a great deal of time sitting, whether it's at a desk, on a plane, or while talking on the phone. Some simple stretches, even once a day, will help get out the kinks, promote better circulation, and help you feel centered and energized.

There are some stretches you can do in bed when you awaken, when you're making your morning smoothie, or even when you're seated at your desk.

Practitioners of yoga say you're only as young as your spine, so a flexible spine is an indicator of a youthful and healthy outlook on life.

Start this week to do the simple routine shown in "Morning Stretches" that moves your spine in all of its six directions. You can do it in five minutes.

MORNING STRETCHES

Up and Down

Stand with your feet shoulder width apart.

Inhale and slowly begin to raise your arms in front of you and straight up over your head.

Stretch as tall as you can.

Breathing deeply, move your arms as if you are climbing a rope, hand over hand.

Keeping your arms over your head, exhale and slowly press your pelvis forward, arching your back and bending backward as far as you comfortably can. Be sure to have your eyes open for this part.

Take a breath or two.

Inhale back to vertical.

On an exhalation, slowly begin to lower your arms and, with your back straight, bend forward and reach toward your toes.

When you've reached down as far as you can, round your back and relax in this forward-bending posture. Breathe deeply. Do not bounce. Hold for about 30 seconds.

With your back rounded, inhale and slowly curl back up to a standing position.

Half Moon

Stand with your feet a little more than shoulder width apart.

Inhaling, raise your arms over your head.

Clasp your hands together over your head.

Exhaling, jut your left hip out, bend straight to your right and bring your body into a crescent moon position. If you are doing this correctly, you'll feel the stretch from the tips of your fingers all the way to your ankles.
Breathe.
Inhale back to vertical and repeat on the other side.

Twist

Sit on the floor with your legs stretched out straight in front of you.
Exhale and bring your left hand behind you on the floor and twist to the left. Bring your right hand to the outside of your left knee.
Breathe.
Inhale and return to the center position.
Repeat in the opposite direction.
Sit quietly for a minute or so.
Note: always move slowly into these stretches, taking your time. Do not bounce or force yourself into the pose.

Be sure to record your breathing and stretching in your Wellness Journal. You may notice some changes even the first day. Keeping close track of your progress will serve as an inspiration in the coming weeks. It'll also help you in your search for the underlying causes of your symptoms, so become a prolific writer and note anything that seems different. As insignificant as something may seem now, a few weeks from now, it may become an important clue.

2

WEEK 2

Self-Evaluation

———

Now it's time to start your detective work by filling out the general health questionnaire. This is similar to the one I use in my office for my patients. It not only gives me insight into what may be going on with them but also allows them to become familiar with my approach.

These are somewhat different from the usual physician questions because they focus on conditions that are body-wide and are not restricted to the individual systems (e.g., cardiovascular or respiratory). You'll be the only one who will read your answers, and, in order to get to the root of your health problems, it's essential for you to be completely honest. Copy these blank pages and put them in your journal. You can also download them from www.drcass.com).

Fill out the entire questionnaire. It's important to do all the sections, even if you think they don't apply to you. You'll notice that some of the same symptoms are involved in several imbalances.

GENERAL HEALTH QUESTIONNAIRE

List your major symptoms: _____

In each of the following sections, put a check mark next to the symptoms that apply to you:

Section 1: Lifestyle and Stress

☐ Difficulty relaxing

☐ Irritability

☐ Insomnia

☐ Tension headaches

☐ Impatience

☐ Sense of isolation from others

☐ Taking on too much responsibility

☐ Difficulty delegating

☐ Recent major life change (marriage, divorce, birth of child, death of close relative, purchase of home, new job, loss of job, etc.)

Section 2: Brain Chemistry

☐ Headaches

☐ Excessive fatigue

☐ Low energy

☐ Weight gain/difficulty losing weight

☐ Memory loss/difficulty concentrating

☐ Sustained high stress level

☐ Nervousness

☐ Depression

☐ Crying easily and often

☐ Anxiety, irritability

Section 3: Sex Hormones

Note all of the symptoms that apply to you within two weeks before your period:

☐ Weight gain

☐ Depression, anxiety, irritability

☐ Sore or swollen breasts

☐ Abdominal bloating or swelling

☐ Lower backache

☐ Craving for sweets

☐ Headaches

☐ Vaginal itching

☐ Recurrent vaginal discharge

☐ Irregular periods

☐ Breast lumps (fibrocystic breasts)

☐ Intensification of other premenstrual syndrome (PMS) symptoms

Note all of the symptoms that apply to you during your period:

☐ Bad cramps ☐ Heavy bleeding

Note all of the symptoms that apply to you if you are experiencing menopause or perimenopause:

☐ Hot flashes, night sweats

☐ Mood swings, irritability

☐ Insomnia

☐ Erratic or missed periods

☐ Dry skin, hair, vagina

☐ Painful intercourse

☐ Known or suspected osteoporosis

☐ Joint pain

☐ Fibromyalgia

☐ Hysterectomy

☐ Loss of interest in sex

Section 4: Thyroid and Adrenals

Thyroid

☐ Excessive fatigue, especially first thing in the morning

☐ Weight gain/difficulty losing weight

☐ Dry skin

☐ Dry, brittle hair

☐ Constipation

☐ Easily chilled; cold and/or numb hands, feet

☐ Forgetfulness

☐ Low sex drive

☐ Depression

☐ Outer third of eyebrow missing or thinning

Low Adrenal Function

☐ Excessive fatigue

☐ Inhalant allergies such as dust, mold, asthma, hay fever

☐ Sensitivity to smog, fumes, and smoke

☐ Trouble falling asleep and, even more, staying asleep

☐ Low blood pressure

☐ Craving for salty foods

☐ Sensitivity to weather changes

☐ Dizziness when standing up suddenly

☐ Dark blue or black circles under eyes

☐ Susceptibility to colds or infections

☐ Puffy and swollen body (water retention)

Section 5: Blood Sugar

Note all of the symptoms from the list that apply to you:

Hypoglycemia

- ☐ Excessive fatigue
- ☐ Dizziness when standing up quickly
- ☐ Irritability, shakiness, or headache with missed meal, relieved by food
- ☐ Craving for sweets
- ☐ Heart palpitations when you eat something sweet

- ☐ Fatigue one to three hours after eating, especially carbs/sweets
- ☐ Use of caffeine to get energy
- ☐ Mood swings
- ☐ Poor concentration
- ☐ Wakefulness during the night with restlessness and worry

Diabetes

- ☐ Extreme thirst
- ☐ Frequent urination
- ☐ Extreme fatigue
- ☐ Night sweats
- ☐ Overweight

- ☐ Frequent infections including yeast infections
- ☐ Family history of diabetes
- ☐ Slow wound healing
- ☐ Numbness or tingling in hands and/or feet

Section 6: Digestive Imbalance Including Dysbiosis, Yeast (Candida), and Food Sensitivities

- ☐ Use of antibiotics for more than one month at any time in your life
- ☐ Recent use of broad-spectrum antibiotics
- ☐ Digestive problems including bloating and gas
- ☐ Cravings for sweets, alcohol, bread, pasta
- ☐ Recurrent vaginal infections
- ☐ Cystitis, interstitial cystitis, or recurring bladder infections

- ☐ General feeling of being tired all over
- ☐ Poor concentration and memory; feeling spacey at times
- ☐ Sensitivity to perfumes, strong smells, tobacco smoke
- ☐ Headaches
- ☐ Muscle aches
- ☐ Pain or swelling in joints
- ☐ Endometriosis or infertility

Section 7: Toxin Overload

☐ Susceptibility to infections

☐ Nausea

☐ Clumsiness

☐ Frequent irritability and anger

☐ Memory loss, which may be intermittent

☐ Irregular heartbeat

☐ Dizziness

☐ Headaches

☐ Tinnitus (ringing in the ears)

☐ Numerous food allergies and/or sensitivities

☐ Unexplained fatigue

Section 8: Headaches, Arthritis, and Osteoporosis

☐ Generalized aches or stiffness

☐ Stiff, painful, or swollen joints

☐ Easy fracture; i.e., brittle bones

☐ Muscle spasms or cramps

☐ Leg cramps at night

☐ Back pain

☐ Bursitis or tendinitis

☐ Neck and shoulder pain

☐ Postmenopausal

☐ Extreme fatigue

Now let's look at your results.

If you've noted three or more symptoms in one category, you can go to the appropriate chapter for more information. It will give you some more clues about the direction you'll need to take to regain your health. Then you will create your action plan based on what you've discovered. This will include food, supplements, activities, and further investigation, including lab tests.

Make a note of the imbalances you are further investigating in your journal entries for Week 2. Here are topics to address:

1. Category or categories in which I checked three items or more on the questionnaire: _____

_____

2. After reading the relevant chapters, these are my insights and thoughts:

_____

_____

_____

3. Based on my newfound information and my intuition, my major imbalance is:

_____

_____

4. The reasons I think this are: _____

_____

_____

_____

Let's return to Kate and Mira.

Kate's questionnaire had high scores in all the hormone categories—thyroid (overweight, tired, and cold), adrenal (tired, dizzy when she stood up suddenly), and sex hormones (PMS). She noticed that she might have a brain chemistry imbalance as well, which would explain her low moods. She recorded all this information and then read the relevant sections.

Kate's educated guess for her most likely problem was hypothyroidism. I agreed. In fact, just her dependence on her morning espresso was a tip-off. Women with low thyroid function have particular trouble getting going in the morning and often use coffee as a wake-me-up. Since low thyroid goes hand in hand with low adrenal function, she'll need to address both, as described in chapter 12.

Mira had already noticed her unbalanced diet. Then, and after reading the material on supplements, we added more essential fatty acids in the form of fish and fish oil capsules. Her questionnaire showed that brain chemistry (low moods and sleep problems) and hormones (sleep problems, irregular periods, and dry skin and hair) were her main issues.

3

WEEK 3

Diagnostic Lab Tests

You'll be pretty busy this week, but please take some time to review your journal entries. The little pearls of insight you've likely had in the past two weeks will provide valuable leads as you continue your search for renewed health.

Be sure to keep up your nutrition, supplement and exercise routines from Week 1, as you will do throughout your entire Vibrant Health Plan. Research shows that it takes three weeks to form a new habit, so this third week is especially important since your good health habits are becoming ingrained. We hope that these new ways of looking at food, nutrition and exercise will become habits that will stay with you for the rest of your life.

Now it's time to do some scientific detective work to back up your suspicions about what's going on with your body. This is exactly what I do in my office. After patients have filled out their questionnaires and I have taken their history, I develop a list of possible imbalances. I then order appropriate lab testing to find out if there is a basis for my suspicions.

Of course, any competent doctor knows that lab testing is no substitute for good overall medical know-how, experience and intuition. We also know that one lab result is not the whole story. These numbers can fluctuate throughout the day or week based on such factors as diet, activities, stress level and where you are in your menstrual cycle. If we get back a result that looks abnormal and doesn't quite fit with the clinical picture, we can always repeat the test for confirmation. In good medical practice, we treat the person, not the lab test!

Do your lab tests as soon as possible because it takes time for your results to come back. It may take anywhere from a few days at a local clinic to a few weeks for mailed-in tests. While you're waiting, you will have enough information to proceed without them, and you can incorporate changes when the results arrive. You may also want to defer testing until later and that's fine, too. Work at your own pace and within your budget.

If you're lucky enough to have a doctor who's willing to join you in the quest for your health, you have won half the battle. You can ask your doctor to order some of the basic, office-based tests and maybe even have them covered by your health insurance.

However, it's not absolutely essential to have a doctor at this point. Many of the lab tests we recommend are available without a prescription. Some are available in community clinics or even in drugstores and supermarkets. Others are available as kits you can purchase at pharmacies. There are some you can do at home—saliva, blood spot (finger prick), urine or hair samples. Others require a drawn blood sample that must be taken by a professional.

We'll give you more information about where to get lab tests as well as about finding supportive doctors in case you need one to order further tests or write prescriptions. Check out the Resources section. You can find out how to order various lab tests online at www.drcass.com.

It's also not necessary to do all of these tests. In my own practice, I generally order a CBC, chemistry panel, lipid panel and liver function panel. Others, such as thyroid and other hormone panels, are ordered only as needed. I frequently order more specific tests, such as organic acid testing, amino acid levels, neurotransmitter levels and stool tests. Look for them at Metametrix Labs(www.metametrix.com), or Genovations (www.gdx.net). These can be costly and are not always covered by insurance. Your test results will give you the general picture of what's happening in your body and where there may be imbalances. Don't forget to refer to any lab results done in the past year or so. You paid for the tests. They're yours. Even if it's been a while, it's useful to have a baseline for comparison.

WHEN YOU GET YOUR RESULTS

Your results will be a series of numbers that may seem confusing, but the important part is that the lab will let you know the normal ranges and where you fall within them. These ranges often come in two categories: the medical norms (averages) and the norms of good health (optimal ranges). The first are average values of the general population, which include people who are not overtly ill but may not be in great health, either. *Optimal ranges* are where you want to be for good health. The specific meanings of *millimoles, milligrams per deciliter,* and other units of measure are essentially unimportant for our purposes here. What you really want to know is whether you fall within the normal and optimal ranges. You'll then focus on the problem areas that fall outside the *optimal* ranges.

Here are the basic tests we suggest you get this week:

BLOOD PRESSURE

Blood pressure is the force of blood against the walls of the arteries. It's recorded as two numbers: the systolic pressure (as the heart beats) and the diastolic pressure (as the heart relaxes between beats).

This is a very simple test. If you're visiting your doctor, someone will likely take your blood pressure. Be sure to ask for your results. You may actually have a blood pressure gauge (called a sphygmomanometer) in your home. If not, many drugstores and even supermarkets have machines to do the testing. You may also be able to get your blood pressure taken by your office nurse, at a health fair or at another free screening.

Try not to take your blood pressure the day your period begins since many women experience harmless blood pressure increases then. Also, you may get a deceptively high reading if you're feeling ill or if you've got a cold or flu. Many people also have what's called white-coat syndrome or elevated blood pressure in a doctor's office but at no other time. If that's the case, it would be a good idea to get your own blood pressure monitor so you can check yourself under relaxed conditions.

You can buy good and simple-to-use monitors at most drug stores. There are also the more expensive (but simpler to use) digital devices that will inflate themselves and then gradually deflate, automatically taking your blood pressure and pulse as they go, and may even give you a printout.

Average blood pressure is not more than 120 mmHg (millimeters of mercury) systolic and 80 mmHg diastolic, and that's what you're looking for. That means the top number is 120 and the bottom number is 80. It's usually expressed as "120 over 80" or "120/80."

Anything above a systolic pressure of 120 may be a cause for concern. However, if you've gotten a high reading, you may want to retest in different circumstances several times to be sure there hasn't been an error.

Conversely, a reading much lower than 120/80 may also be a cause for concern. I can't count the number of patients who have come to me believing the myth of low blood pressure. They've been congratulated by a doctor or nurse for having low blood pressure, say 100/70. The truth is, they are chronically tired, and feel dizzy when they stand up quickly. *Rather than meaning they are "extra healthy," low blood pressure for them is a likely sign of low adrenal function.*

Enter your blood pressure reading in your Wellness Journal.

RESTING PULSE

You'll also want to know your resting pulse rate. It's easy to take it yourself:

Sit quietly for at least two minutes.

Firmly place the index finger and middle finger on the opposite wrist, in line with the large thumb muscle.

Find your pulse.

Count beats for 10 seconds.

Multiply by six.

This is your resting pulse rate.

Normal resting pulse ranges are generally between 65 and 80 unless you are a highly conditioned athlete, in which case your resting pulse may be lower. If your resting pulse is under 60, it could also be a sign of low adrenal function.

CHOLESTEROL AND TRIGLYCERIDE SCREENING

Cholesterol is a waxy, fatlike substance that occurs naturally in all parts of the body and is essential for normal body function. Cholesterol is present in cell walls and membranes everywhere in your body, including the brain, nerves, muscle, skin, liver, intestines and heart. Your body needs cholesterol to produce such components as hormones, brain cells, vitamin D and the bile acids that help digest fat.

Conventional medicine says that excess cholesterol is deposited in the arteries, where it contributes to the formation of artery-clogging plaque, increasing the risk of heart attack and stroke. In fact, the cholesterol forms in response to inflammation in the vessel wall, so the focus should be more on treating the source of the inflammation than on eating less fat.

While eating foods high in saturated fat and cholesterol can raise your blood cholesterol, the rise is generally temporary and does not usually contribute to plaque formation. The real culprit is excessive intake of refined carbohydrates such as sugar and white flour which cause an inflammatory response, in the form of raised cholesterol. Fat cells themselves (adipocytes) are source of inflammation, accounting for elevated cholesterol in obese individuals.

HDL (high-density lipoprotein) or "good" cholesterol helps clear arteries of fat and cholesterol, carrying it to the liver for removal from the body. LDL (low-density lipoprotein) or "bad" cholesterol deposits cholesterol on your arterial walls and causes them to become clogged

Triglycerides are the fats in your blood, derived from fats eaten in foods or made by your body from other energy sources, such as carbohydrates. The calories you eat that are not used for immediate energy needs are converted to triglycerides and sent to fat cells for storage.

High triglycerides may be a sign of undiagnosed diabetes or low thyroid, and they may reflect an increased risk for heart disease.

Blood cholesterol and triglycerides are usually checked by a simple blood test, available through your doctor, at community screening clinics and health fairs, and through consumer labs (i.e., those not requiring a prescription from your doctor). To get accurate results, you'll need to refrain from eating and drinking anything but water for about 10 hours before the blood is drawn. Your cholesterol measurement will be given in three numbers: total cholesterol, HDL and LDL cholesterol.

You're aiming for total cholesterol of less than 200 mg/dL. Here are the ranges:

Normal: 200 mg/dL or less
Borderline-high cholesterol: 200–239 mg/dL

High risk for heart disease: 240 mg/dL or more
Optimal total cholesterol range: 180–200

HDL cholesterol which protects against heart disease should be between 60 and 150 mg/dL. The higher your HDL cholesterol, the better you are assimilating fats in your system. Below 40 mg/dL is inadequate.

LDL (bad) cholesterol levels: The goal is to keep these levels low.
Optimal is below 100 mg/dL
Near optimal is 100–129
High is 160–189
Very high is 190 and above

When looking at your total cholesterol levels, the ratio is more important than the numbers, with an optimal ratio of total cholesterol to HDL at 3:1 or less. Normal range is considered 5:1 or less.

Most conventional doctors have been led to believe that very low total cholesterol is the way to go. Your doctor may prescribe cholesterol-lowering medication called statins but they are not the only solution. Some standards even mandate total cholesterol levels that are impossible to achieve without the use of statin drugs. However, these drugs pose a hazard to your health and there is simply no research that proves they protect against heart attacks. The reason is simple: These so-called cholesterol-lowering drugs don't address the causes of plaque in arteries. Here are some facts that you may not know:
Here are some statin facts that you may not know:

- A review of five big studies found that the risk of non-fatal heart attack and stroke was reduced by 1.4% in people on statin therapy—but that the rate of serious adverse effects *rose* 1.8% in those same people. Not a great trade-off.

- There is no relationship between blood cholesterol and heart disease risk in women over fifty or in men over seventy. Statins given to these individuals are not only wasted, but expose them to risk of side effects that isn't outweighed by benefit to their hearts.

- A survey of South Carolina adults found no correlation of blood cholesterol levels with "bad" dietary habits, such as use of red meat, animal fats, fried foods, butter, eggs, whole milk, bacon, sausage, and cheese.

- A Medical Research Council survey showed that men eating butter ran half the risk of developing heart disease compared with those using margarine.

- Mother's milk provides a higher proportion of cholesterol than almost any other food. It also contains over 50% of its calories as fat, much of it saturated fat. Both cholesterol and saturated fat are essential for growth in babies and children, especially for the development of the brain. Yet, the American Heart Association is now recommending that children consume a low-cholesterol, low-fat diet. That's exactly the kind of diet that was linked, in one recent study, with failure to thrive in children. The fact is, children need good fats to provide the raw materials for healthy brain cells.

Statins *have* been found to help with heart attack and stroke prevention in two groups of people: Those with type 2 diabetes and those who have already had a heart attack or stroke and want to prevent another one. The catch is that the drugs probably don't help these people because they lower cholesterol, but because they address another, more important risk factor: inflammation.

Pardon this seeming diversion, but statins are overprescribed, and often not worth the risk of their side effects.

Your triglyceride results can be evaluated as follows:

Normal: less than 150 mg/dLBorderline high: 150–199 mg/dL
High: 200–499 mg/dL
Very high: 500 mg/dL or higher

If you are concerned about your cholesterol levels being too high and the implications for your cardiovascular health, there are two other markers for you to consider:

To test for inflammation, get a *quantitative* C-reactive protein level. Optimal levels should be 0.7 or less. Normal is up to 2.

Also, high levels of an amino acid called homocysteine, a harmful by-product of protein metabolism, have been associated with heart disease, stroke and Alzheimer's disease. Optimal level is less than 9. If it's elevated, you are probably deficient in the essential vitamins such as vitamins B_{12}, B_6 and folic acid, and you'll need to supplement with them.

For a more detailed explanation, including interpretation of lab tests, you can go to such sites as www.webmd.com.

COMPREHENSIVE METABOLIC PANEL

The Comprehensive Metabolic Panel (CMP) is typically a group of 14 specific blood tests that have been approved, named, and assigned a CPT code (Current Procedural Terminology number) by Medicare, and most insurance companies. It is performed on the blood serum (the portion of blood without cells). Here is what it measures, with the normal ranges:

Glucose level is a measure of how well the body is converting carbohydrates into energy and how well the liver and other organs that help regulate blood sugar are working. Measured fasting, i.e. 9–12 hours after the last meal, elevated blood glucose levels can indicate diabetes, liver disease, hypothyroidism, or stress-related illnesses. Low levels are a sign of hypoglycemia. Normal range is 65–109 mg/dL. (Optimal is 70–100.). If blood glucose is abnormally high or low, I will order a HbA1C or glycosylated hemoglobin, which more accurately measures an average level of glucose over time. Normal range: 4.0–5.9%. Under that reflects hypoglycemia, while above that range, diabetes.

Kidney Function

Blood urea nitrogen (BUN) measures the amount of nitrogen in your blood derived from urea, which is formed in the liver as a byproduct of protein metabolism. The kidneys then eliminate urea in the urine. Elevated levels can indicate kidney disease. It can also reflect heart disease, dehydration, or excessive protein intake. Liver disease can lead to a low BUN.

Normal range is 7–20 mg/dL.

Creatinine is a breakdown product of creatine, a constituent of muscle, and measures the kidneys' ability to excrete waste in the urine. Elevated creatinine levels can indicate kidney problems. Normal range is .8–1.4 mg/dL.

Total protein measurements can reflect nutritional status, kidney disease, liver disease, and many other conditions. Normal range is 6.5–8.0 g/100ml.

Albumin is the major protein in the blood. Low albumin is generally a sign of liver or kidney problems. Normal range is 3.4–5.4 g/dL

Electrolytes

The concentrations of sodium and potassium are tightly regulated by the body as is the balance between these four elements. Electrolyte (and acid-base) imbalances can be present in a wide variety of acute and chronic illnesses.

Serum chloride shows the amount of chloride in the blood serum and it's often related to changes in sodium levels. Elevated serum chloride can indicate dehydration, diarrhea or conditions causing excessive urination. Low levels can indicate kidney disease, uncontrolled diabetes, congestive heart failure, cirrhosis of the liver, very high protein, triglycerides or glucose in the blood. Normal range is 101–111 mmol/L.

Serum sodium shows the amount of sodium in the serum and is linked to serum chloride. Elevated levels can be a risk factor for hypertension, while low levels often reflect low adrenal function, which is more common than most people realize. Normal range is 136–144 mEq/L.

Carbon dioxide (CO_2) determines the amount of carbon dioxide in your blood, which indicates how well your kidneys and lungs are controlling the acid-base balance in your body. Excessive or depressed levels can indicate kidney problems, breathing or lung problems, poisoning or drug overdose, severe diarrhea, uncontrolled diabetes or severe dehydration. Normal range is 20–29 mmol/L.

Serum potassium measures blood levels of potassium which is essential to proper heart function. Elevated potassium can indicate kidney problems or dehydration. Low levels can be caused by severe vomiting or diarrhea, the use of diuretics or liver disease. Normal range is 3.5–5.5 mEq/L.

Calcium is one of the most important minerals in your body. Blood calcium is tested to screen for a range of conditions relating to the bones, heart, nerves, kidneys, and teeth. Normal range is 8.5 to 10.2 mg/dL

LIVER FUNCTION PANEL

The liver is the largest organ in the body, weighing around 3.5 pounds. It has a major role in the metabolism, digestion, detoxification, and elimination of various potentially toxic substances from the body. A liver panel will show

how healthy this major organ is by measuring levels of various enzymes that it produces:

AST (aspartate aminotransferase) was formerly called SGOT (serum glutamic-oxaloacetic transaminase). Normal range is 9–72 U/L.

ALT (alanine aminotransferase) was formerly called SGPT (serum glutamic-pyruvic transaminase). Normal range is 8–50 U/L. Both enzymes are elevated in cases of liver cell damage. Both are also found in myocardial cells (heart muscle) and skeletal muscle cells. AST is also in bone, and ALT is in the kidneys. Liver damage from alcohol, various diseases, strenuous exercise, and various prescription drugs can lead to elevated results in either one.

Bilirubin is a breakdown product of hemoglobin from red blood cells. Total bilirubin and direct bilirubin are usually measured for screening and/or monitoring liver or gallbladder problems. Normal range is .2–1.3 mg/dL.

ALP (alkaline phosphatase) is an enzyme made mostly in liver and bone, and is elevated when the body tissue is diseased. Increased ALP levels can also be due to medications and healing of fractures. Normal range is 38–126 U/L.

LDH (lactate dehydrogenase) is an enzyme that helps produce energy. Found in the kidneys, liver, heart, muscle, brain, lungs and red blood cells, it is raised when there is injury; for example, 24–48 hrs after a heart attack. Normal range is. 105–330 IU/liter.

COMPLETE BLOOD COUNT (CBC)

The complete blood count (CBC) measures five major components of blood:

White blood cell count (WBC) measures your ability to fight infections. Normal range is 3.4–9.6 K/mm.

Red blood cell count (RBC) measures the number of red blood cells that carry oxygen and remove waste products from body tissues. Normal range is 3.58–4.99 mil/mm^3. (Optimal is 3.8–5.1 for women.)

Hemoglobin (HGB) value measures your body's ability to carry oxygen to tissues and remove carbon dioxide from tissues to lungs. Hemoglobin gives the red color to blood. Normal range is 11.1–15.0 g/dL. (Optimal level is upper range of normal.)

Hematocrit (HCT) value measures the percentage of red blood cells in relation to your total blood volume. Normal range is 31.8–43.2%. (Optimal range is upper end of normal.)

Platelet count measures your ability to stop bleeding by forming clots. Normal range in a complete blood count is 140–440 K/mm^3. (Optimal is 162–380.)

Among other things, your CBC will let you know if you are anemic, which is a major cause of fatigue that can be due to a deficiency in iron, folic acid, B_{12}, or B_6. A high white blood cell count is due to infection, inflammation, or, if very high, leukemia or other more serious conditions. A low WBC may indicate immune-system impairment.

White blood cells are divided further into six main types: neutrophils (elevated in bacterial infections, inflammation, etc.), bands (new neutrophils, in response to an acute bacterial infection), lymphocytes (further divided into T- and B-lymphocytes, and elevated in viral and chronic infections), basophils (decreased in acute allergic reactions), eosinophils (elevated in allergy or parasites), and monocytes (elevated in viral infection, inflammation).

These are the normal relative values of each:

- Neutrophils: 40 to 60%
- Bands: 0 to 3%
- Lymphocytes: 20 to 40%
- Basophils: 0.5 to 1%
- Eosinophils: 1 to 4%
- Monocytes: 2 to 8%

The tests are done by drawing a small test tube full of blood. This can be the same tube as the blood for your cholesterol screening, so you don't have to have your skin punctured twice for the blood draw.

These are the basic tests. More specific testing will be found in the imbalances chapters. If you know what blood tests you want to have done, make a list and do them all at once for convenience.

Breast Self-Exam

The value of breast self-exams has recently been questioned, with some experts saying that it is difficult to teach women to do a comprehensive exam. We think women are intelligent enough to seek and find problems in their breasts. In addition, women often intuitively know when something is wrong.

The breast self-exam is a simple procedure that takes less than five minutes a month—and it could save your life. If you find a lump, check with your doctor. While only about 15 to 20% of lumps turn out to be malignant, it's better to be safe than sorry. For more details, see www.breastcancer.org.

While conventional doctors are very focused on mammograms as preventive and diagnostic tools, there are safer alternatives. The average mammogram exposes a woman to100 times the radiation of a chest X-ray. We know that radiation causes cancer, so it makes no sense to use radiation to screen for cancer. The compression caused by the mammogram machine may also cause existing lumps to "leak" malignant cells.

Thermograms are an excellent non-invasive alternative to mammograms that can actually provide more information. Thermograms cost about the same as mammograms and can warn you years earlier than mammograms if abnormal tissues growth is beginning. That being said, it requires an expert to interpret and there have been occasional cases of false negatives, i.e. missed tumors, with thermograms.

For more information on thermograms and other means of keeping your breasts healthy, please see *The Secret of Health: Breast Wisdom* which Kathleen Barnes wrote with Dr. Ben Johnson. (Morgan James 2008)

WEIGHT/BODY FAT

You can use your bathroom scale or, for a little more money, get one that will assess body fat percentages as well as weight.

You will need to calculate what is called your BMI or body mass index, the ratio between your height and weight.

An excellent chart for BMI calculation can be found on the website: www.consumer.gov/weightloss/bmi.htm.

Here's what your BMI means:

    17–19: underweight

    20–24: normal

    25–29: overweight

    30–39: obese

    40 and up: extremely obese

Body fat percentages can be tested in a number of ways, but the simplest and most common involves the use of a pair of calipers that measures the thickness of skin folds. Many personal trainers at gyms have these instruments. The most high-tech way of measuring percent lean mass versus body weight is with a bio-electric impedance device, found in some gyms and clinics. For women, an acceptable range of body fat is 25% or less. The proportion of fat to lean body mass is more important than weight or even than looking thin. There are thin

BMI (KG/M²)	19	20	21	22	23	24	25	26	27	28	29	30	35	40
HEIGHT (IN.)							WEIGHT (LB.)							
58	91	96	100	105	110	115	119	124	129	134	138	143	167	191
59	94	99	104	109	114	119	124	128	133	138	143	148	173	198
60	97	102	107	112	118	123	128	133	138	143	148	153	179	204
61	100	106	111	116	122	127	132	137	143	148	153	158	185	211
62	104	109	115	120	126	131	136	142	147	153	158	164	191	218
63	107	113	118	124	130	135	141	146	152	158	163	169	197	225
64	110	116	122	128	134	140	145	151	157	163	169	174	204	232
65	114	120	126	132	138	144	150	156	162	168	174	180	210	240
66	118	124	130	136	142	148	155	161	167	173	179	186	216	247
67	121	127	134	140	146	153	159	166	172	178	185	191	223	255
68	125	131	138	144	151	158	164	171	177	184	190	197	230	262
69	128	135	142	149	155	162	169	176	182	189	196	203	236	270
70	132	139	146	153	160	167	174	181	188	195	202	207	243	278
71	136	143	150	157	165	172	179	186	193	200	208	215	250	286
72	140	147	154	162	169	177	184	191	199	206	213	221	258	294
73	144	151	159	166	174	182	189	197	204	212	219	227	265	302
74	148	155	163	171	179	186	194	202	210	218	225	233	272	311
75	152	160	168	176	184	192	200	208	216	224	232	240	279	319
76	156	164	172	180	189	197	205	213	221	230	238	246	287	328

Body weight in pounds according to height and body mass index.

women with too much fat (including many anorexics!), and there are large women who have the correct proportion of fat to muscle.

Waist-to-hip ratio is another good number to know. You will learn about Metabolic Syndrome later, but suffice it to say for now, excessive abdominal fat (an apple-shaped figure as opposed to a pear-shaped figure) represents a higher risk for heart disease, diabetes, and some types of cancer. Here's how to determine waist-hip ratio:

Measure your waist and hips, and then divide the hip measurement by the waist measurement. In women, a ratio of .8 is an indicator for obesity-related diseases.

FLEXIBILITY/FITNESS

These are fairly subjective tests, but as a rule, for absolute minimum fitness you should be able to do the following:

- Touch your toes with your knees straight, without bouncing.

- Slowly lift a 10-pound weight from the floor to over your head. Repeat as many times as you can. You should be able to repeat at least 10 times without exhaustion.

- Walk a mile in 20 minutes or less with your finishing heart rate under 180. You should return to your resting pulse within 10 minutes.

YOUR WELLNESS JOURNAL WORK SHEET

As you get your test results, whether from a lab or from something you've done for yourself, record them in your Wellness Journal.

Note: Many laboratories use different units of measure in their testing, so don't be surprised if you get results that are different from the ones we gave. There is also the "average" versus the "optimal" value. Your test results should come with the normal ranges your lab uses and, with those that work directly with consumers, an explanation. Many labs will not include optimal values. Here's a sample work sheet you can copy and insert in your journal. Put a mark next to any result that is outside the normal ranges.

MY TEST RESULTS

Basic Tests

	MY READING	NORMAL RANGE
Blood pressure		120/80 mmHg
Resting pulse		65–80
Total cholesterol		200mg/dL or less
HDL cholesterol		60 mg/dL or higher
LDL cholesterol		under 100 mg/dL
Triglycerides		150 mg/dL or less

Liver Function Panel

	MY READING	NORMAL RANGE
AST		9–72 U/L
ALT		8–50 U/L
Bilirubin		.2–1.3 mg/dL
ALP		38–126 U/L
LDH		105–333 IU/L

CBC

	MY READING	NORMAL RANGE
White cell count		3.4–9.6 K/mm³
Red cell count		3.58–4.99 mil/mm³
Hemoglobin		11.1–15.0 g/dL
Hematocrit		31.8–43.2%
Platelets		140–440 K/mm³

Comprehensive Metabolic Panel (CMP)

	MY READING	NORMAL RANGE
Blood urea nitrogen (BUN)		7–20 mg/dL
Serum chloride		101–111 mmol/L
Serum sodium		136–144 mEq/L
Carbon dioxide (CO_2)		20–29 mmol/L
Creatinine		.8–1.4 mg/dL
Glucose		65–109 mg/dL
Serum potassium		3.5–5.5 mEq/L

Weight/Body Fat

	MY READING	NORMAL RANGE
Body mass index		under 25
Body fat		25% or less
Waist-hip ratio		.8 or less

What I've learned from these tests: _____

_____

_____

Make notes in your journal of your general thoughts about which imbalances you are experiencing.

As we said at the beginning of this chapter, it may take longer than a week for you to order your tests, complete them, and get your results back. The time this takes also depends on which tests you decide to do. The assignment this week was to get the ball rolling, not to finish everything, so if you've started, you're doing just great.

Your exercise and deep-breathing programs are probably making you feel better already. Keep it up! If you had an indulgence here and there, don't worry, just pick up your Vibrant Health Plan where you left off. And do give yourself a pat on the back for all the *good* things you are doing for yourself. We are often self-critical about our failings and forget to reward ourselves for our positive actions.

Remember: You're in charge of your health. You are making great strides toward bringing yourself back to the glowing health you deserve.

Soon you'll have all the the tools you need to make some solid decisions about where to look for the cause of your health problems.

4

WEEK 4

Making Your Plan

———

Now is the time for you to take what you've learned about your health so far and use that information to discover the underlying imbalances that are the source of your health problems.

You know the major health complaints you will be working on.

You've made some basic changes to your diet, sleep, and exercise patterns and you're probably already beginning to see some results.

The questionnaires and the testing you've now completed will provide some concrete information about how to figure out the underlying imbalances. You may not yet have received all of your lab results, but you can go ahead with this chapter anyway. You can always revise your plan if results come in future weeks that change your focus.

Review all your research now. It will clarify which direction you should take. This process is going to be part science, part intuition, and a good part just common sense.

We women grow up in a world where our intuition is not necessarily respected by others, and sometimes we lose trust in our own "knowing." As women, both of us have learned over the years to trust our own intuition and to honor it in others. It sure helps me in diagnosing and treating patients. But you don't have to be a doctor to trust your intuition.

While she is not a trained medical professional, Kathleen, has worked with the spiritual aspects of healing for most of her adult life and is well acquainted with intuitive medicine and energetic healing.

We all have innate healing ability that we use most easily with our children and other loved ones. How about using it on yourself now?

Let's begin with a unique and intuitive means of discovering what your innate wisdom sees as helpful for you. This will be a valuable tool for this week's decision making.

CONTACTING YOUR HIGHER INTELLIGENCE

Do you ever hear a still, small voice inside? It's the one that you may override and then later discover gave your correct information all along. We sure have! Both of us have learned to rely on the little voice, even though our professional colleagues might think that "hearing voices" is a little strange. It works!

For me, the little voice has communicated everything from such mundane messages as "Take your sweater. You'll need it," to "Check that patient for copper toxicity" (honestly!).

For the most part, the voice turns out to be right. At times, it may tell you to stop in at a particular place, and if you're tuned in enough to listen, you end up running into someone you had wanted to see or had been thinking of. This same voice has higher octaves as well—messages you receive about your life path—when you allow yourself the time and quiet to listen to it.

The voice may sound like your own, so you can't simply assume that it's someone out there watching over you (though it might be). It's sometimes just in the form of an idea, an urge or an inspiration.

Whatever we call it and however we imagine it, we all have a helpful inner guide that acts as a compass for us, if only we get quiet enough to listen. Use this voice to help you make your decisions, not just here for your health issues, but in life in general.

Regular meditation will help you get closer to that inner source.

The Decision Tree

Now is the time for you to choose which pathway you will follow for the next six weeks. Take some time to study the table called the "Decision Tree" and locate your most likely imbalances. Then read the information on those imbalances that follows.

Decision Tree

PROBLEM	POSSIBLE IMBALANCE
Fatigue/sleep disturbance	Brain chemistry
	Lifestyle/stress
	Thyroid/adrenal
	Toxin
	Candida/food allergy
Mood (depression, anxiety)	Brain chemistry
	Sex hormone
	Thyroid/adrenal
	Lifestyle/stress
	Toxin
Women's reproductive (PMS, perimenopause, menopause)	Sex hormones
	Thyroid/adrenal
	Lifestyle/stress
	Toxin
	Candida/food allergy
Weight gain*	Thyroid/adrenal
	Blood sugar
	Lifestyle/stress
	Brain chemistry
	Toxin
	Sex hormone
Allergies	Toxin
	Thyroid/adrenal
	Candida/food allergy
Pain	Brain chemistry (headache)
	Lifestyle/stress (headache)
Mental function	Brain chemistry
	Lifestyle/stress
	Sex hormone

If weight issues are high on your symptom list, also read Chapter 17.

THE IMBALANCES

Once you read through these synopses of the possible imbalances, you'll be ready to delve more deeply into the specific chapters in Part 2. As you read through these brief descriptions, you may find that more than one imbalance may be affecting your health. By reading the pertinent chapters, you may get more clarity. As we've said before, all our body systems are interconnected and an imbalance in one often affects other systems. Conversely, correcting an imbalance in one system will often take care of problems elsewhere.

In the chapters in Part 2, each problem listed here will have a brief summary of the conventional medical approach followed by a detailed description of more natural approaches to correcting your imbalances.

Lifestyle and Stress Imbalances

Unresolved stress in your life can lead to a downward spiral that can cause a wide range of physical problems from headaches and heart disease to gastrointestinal problems and more. You will learn to incorporate stress reduction into your life. It's essential!

Brain Chemistry Imbalances

Unbalanced brain chemicals can cause everything from anxiety and insomnia to depression, addiction, memory loss, mood swings and even serious mental illness. You will learn natural ways to correct these imbalances at the root of the problem.

Hormone Imbalances

A hormone is a chemical messenger secreted by any one of the body's endocrine (ductless) glands—the thyroid (thyroid hormone), parathyroid (parathormone), ovaries (estrogen, progesterone), testes (testosterone), adrenals (adrenaline, cortisol, DHEA) and pancreas (insulin).

Sex Hormone Imbalances

As women, we know the feelings associated with hormone swings, whether during our menstrual cycles or when hormone production begins to decline with age, a period known as "perimenopause." Eventually, all of us will experience the hormonal challenges of menopause. There are ways to minimize, even eliminate, symptoms of PMS and menopause by knowing how to balance your hormones.

Thyroid and Adrenal Imbalances

The thyroid and adrenal glands control energy production and when they are out of balance, you'll feel exhausted, possibly depressed and be subject to illness and infection. Mainstream medicine is just not up to speed when it comes to recognizing and treating these increasingly common problems, but we'll give you ways to detect and relieve these imbalances.

Blood Sugar Imbalances and Metabolic Syndrome X

Symptoms of blood sugar imbalance may include low blood sugar (hypoglycemia) and what may seem like its opposite, diabetes, with its high blood sugar. You will learn how these conditions relate to each other and the role that high-sugar foods, insulin and blood sugar levels play in making you feel weak, light-headed or irritable. Correcting your diet is the first line of defense here.

Digestion, Dysbiosis, and Food Allergies

Dysbiosis refers to an imbalance in the normal intestinal bacteria where there is an overgrowth of harmful yeast and other pathogenic organisms or "bad bugs in your gut." They produce toxins that cause all kinds of problems, such as depression, headaches, PMS, chronic fatigue syndrome, allergies, and even asthma.

Multiple food and chemical sensitivities are strongly linked to yeast overgrowth, possibly because the dysbiosis causes imbalances in the immune system. You will learn to detect and eliminate these, as well as the yeast, and restore your digestive and body balance.

Toxin Imbalances

In our modern world, most of us are subject to toxic overloads caused by every-

thing from air pollution to contaminated food and to plastics in our environment to exposure to cigarette smoke. Even generally healthy foods such as fish
can be a source of toxic mercury and poisoning can cause brain and nervous
system damage. Learn how to avoid these toxins and to clear out those already
ingested.

Musculoskeletal Imbalances
(Headaches, Arthritis, and Osteoporosis)

When your body's structure—the bones and muscles that support you—
becomes imbalanced, it can show up as back pain, joint pain, carpal tunnel
syndrome, pinched nerves or headaches. There are methods to detect and
repair the underlying problems rather than simply treating the pain itself.

YOUR NEXT STEP

Now that you've worked your way through your symptoms, the tests and the
relationships among symptoms and imbalances in this chapter, you're ready to
make a choice.

Go to the chapter on the imbalance you consider most likely to be the
underlying cause of your health problem. Then read it carefully and determine
if it applies to you and to your condition. If you have identified more than one
imbalance, use your intuition to pick one to work on first.

If you're still uncertain which imbalance to address first, read through all
the sections that seem to pertain to you, for clarity. Remember that very few
health conditions fit neatly into little slots, so what you see there may not be an
exact fit.

Here is an example of how the various conditions are connected. Despite the
complexity at first glance, the solutions may be surprisingly simple.

Ginny's Story

Twenty-eight-year-old Ginny had graduated from college a few months earlier
and was one month into a demanding new job. She came to me complaining
of recurring headaches and she was 20 pounds overweight. She craved sugary

food and pasta, was tired especially in the late afternoon and had difficulty concentrating. She noticed gas and bloating after meals, as well.

My thoughts?

Her low energy was likely due to blood sugar imbalances.

Low thyroid was another consideration, because she was tired and overweight. Her mother was, too, and had been on thyroid medication at one point in her life. This family history of hypothyroidism was a weak spot in Ginny's armor.

Suggestive of intestinal yeast problems, her bloating had been a longstanding problem, ever since she had taken a six-month course of antibiotics for acne in her teens. Her digestion was worse since she started her new job, too. And her eating habits? Don't ask. No breakfast, coffee and doughnuts at the office, a sandwich at her desk. You get the picture. It was clear too that stress was likely playing a big role in her condition.

Now, is Ginny just an unlucky young woman with myriad health problems, or is she suffering from a basic imbalance that is affecting the rest of her systems?

The fact is, her problems are all interrelated and will begin to resolve once she attacks the likeliest basic cause. Ginny's story is pretty typical for women I see and treat successfully. You can even treat yourself successfully in such a situation once you have read the book and worked with the program.

In a nutshell: In adolescence, Ginny's acne was treated with antibiotics, which killed her gut flora (the "good bugs" that help with digestion), creating a fertile field for yeast. Her stress-driven sugar intake then allowed the yeast to thrive (yeast *loves* sugar!). In addition, her chronic stress weakened her adrenals and drove her blood sugar down, increasing her sweet cravings even further. The yeast also led to "leaky gut" and poor absorption of nutrients, which were needed to run every aspect of her body and brain chemistry. Now, there was a vicious cycle!

Ginny was overweight and undernourished. That's a fairly common combination. This lack of nutrients led to a host of other problems that we haven't even mentioned. For example, one result of her malnutrition was that it deprived her thyroid of the minerals zinc and selenium that it needed to make thyroid hormone. Her acne may have been due to a zinc deficiency in the first place! The result? She was tired and overweight and prone to infections, such as the yeast. So, get the picture? And I didn't even mention her PMS, another by-product of poor diet, low thyroid, stress, and yeast.

Far from a hopeless case, Ginny simply needed to pay attention to exactly the same issues that you will in the course of reading this book. Did it take me hours to figure this out as she sat there? No. It took me longer to write Ginny's story (about 30 minutes) than it did to understand her situation.

You'll get it, too. We are dealing with a multidimensional system: All your body systems relate to each other. The larger picture can be perceived quite easily by the trained eye and the untrained eye just needs some education.

Ginny began to learn about the impact on her health of her lifestyle—food, supplements, exercise, and relaxation. She was actually excited to find out that there was a name to her condition and that she could help fix it. Her core issues? Unbalanced diet, malnutrition, hypothyroidism, intestinal yeast (candida) and unbalanced hormones. The solution? Attack on all fronts!

This is what I recommended for Ginny:

Change diet to nutritious foods.

- Add nutrients (multivitamin and antioxidants), probiotics and antifungal herbal formula.

- Remove sugar and caffeine, which was easier once she had introduced more nourishing foods and supplements.

- Support the adrenals (stressed) with adaptogens and B vitamins.

- Nourish her thyroid with minerals, seaweed, and tyrosine.

- Exercise: To get her metabolism going, gradually, I recommended walking in nature, using the stairs at work, doing yoga or another more meditative form of exercise, getting in touch with her body in the process.

- Meditate.

See how this works? We take many factors into consideration—including the results of your lab tests—and rank them from "most likely" to "least likely." You may already have a pretty good handle on what's going on. Don't worry if it takes some repetition for you to catch on; it has taken me years to integrate all this information, and I'm still learning!

5

WEEK 5

Balance Your Diet

———

"Let food be your medicine."
—HIPPOCRATES

This week you'll be implementing the recommendations for the condition you're addressing. Your imbalance section may include additional questionnaires to help you gain insight into your condition, recommendations for more supplements, dietary changes, increased or different exercise and various other therapies. It may even recommend that you see a doctor.

This chapter will give you an in-depth look at the food issue: You are what you eat and we don't all eat as well as we should. So you will likely be handling your "condition" as well as learning all about food and vitamin supplements.

Please don't add stress to your life by trying to do everything at once. You'll be much more likely to adhere to your new program if you take things at a moderate pace. This is another place to use your intuition about what will work for you.

This week would be a good time to read through your Wellness Journal again, to remind yourself how far you've come in just five short weeks. Re-reading your journal may also trigger some insights that will be helpful in the weeks to come. By this time, you are probably noticing some wonderful changes in your body, mind, and spirit as a result of the basic programs you started in Week 1. Keep up those programs as you continue forward.

FOOD, GLORIOUS FOOD

It's time to start thinking of food as fuel. In order to function at peak efficiency, your body needs the best raw materials possible. Our standard American Diet (SAD for short!), which emphasizes high-fat, high-calorie, low-nutrient eating, is anything but nourishing. We live in a time when food is more plentiful than it has ever been in history, yet we are woefully undernourished because we fill up on all the wrong foods. Many of us eat too many processed foods that have almost no nutritional value. They are high in chemicals, salt, starch and, above all, sugar. It's amazing that our bodies can glean the basic minimum requirements, and often, they don't. That's why even the medical establishment has recognized the need for all adults to take a multivitamin every day.

Depressed, tired, foggy-brained, overweight women are often told they need Prozac, when in fact all they really need is a steady supply of real food to get their brains and bodies back on track. Haven't there been times when you found yourself feeling tired, irritable, unable to think straight, and over-whelmed with all that you had to do—when you suddenly realized that you'd skipped a meal? Within minutes of eating a carrot, a muffin or a piece of cheese, everything changes: the world becomes a better place, and those tasks are no longer insurmountable. The problem was simply low blood sugar: Your poor brain was running on empty!

The next step is to choose the highest-quality food possible to help keep your neurotransmitters in balance.

There is scientific proof that if you follow the principles of optimum nutrition, you can do all of the following:

- Improve your mood.
- Increase your mental and physical stamina and your overall health.
- Enhance your concentration, memory and overall mental ability.
- Reduce your stress level.

In this chapter, we'll be looking at each of the various nutrients from the fuel-supplying carbohydrates to the building-block proteins and fats to the catalysts and cofactors, vitamins and minerals. We'll finish with a list of the basics that will get you, and keep you, in vibrant health.

THE BASIC THREE: CARBOHYDRATE, PROTEIN, AND FAT

All foods fall into one of three categories: carbohydrate, protein, or fat. Our bodies need high-quality versions of all three for optimal health. An excellent dietary mix is to obtain about 40% of your calories from complex carbohydrates, 30% from high-quality protein, and 30% from good fats. If you've cleaned up your diet and you're still experiencing cravings for sugar, caffeine, nicotine, alcohol or recreational drugs, see Chapter 6 for more ways to address these issues.

Weight management is such an important concern for many women that we've included a special bonus chapter, Chapter 17, full of ideas and suggestions to help you get your weight where you want it.

We'll begin with whole foods, which grow in the ground or on trees. They are natural and have undergone little or no processing. They include beans, lentils, seeds, nuts, whole grains such as brown rice, whole wheat bread or pasta, as well as fresh fruit and vegetables. Seeds are especially rich in fiber and in essential minerals like calcium, magnesium, zinc and iron.

Running on Carbohydrates

Your body's main fuel is glucose or blood sugar. Most carbohydrates, including bread, cereals, fruits and vegetables, break down into this simple sugar during digestion. This does not mean that you should eat more sugar to enhance your energy! Quite the opposite. The quick-release sugars found in white flour, candy, cookies, and fruit juices will lead only to the "sugar blues," a sugar high caused by the availability of the quick energy sugars followed by a blood sugar crash. You want a steady supply of glucose for fuel based on complex carbs. Think whole grain toast instead of a Snickers bar.

The speed at which a specific food breaks down into glucose determines its glycemic index (GI). In a nutshell, the higher a food's glycemic index, the more quickly it breaks down into simple sugars and the worse it is for you. However, it's a little more complicated than that for a couple of reasons:

1. Glycemic index or GI tells you only how rapidly a particular carbohydrate turns into sugar. It doesn't tell you how much of that carbohydrate is in a serving of a particular food. You need to know both things to understand a food's effect on blood sugar. That is where glycemic load or GL comes in. The carbohydrate in watermelon, for example, has a high GI. But there isn't a lot of it, so watermelon's glycemic load is relatively low. A GL of 20 or more is high, a GL of 11 through 19 is medium, and a GL of 10 or less is low. Foods that have a low GL almost always have a low GI. Foods with an intermediate or high GL range from very low to very high GI.

2. Glycemic index is based on eating that food alone, something we don't do very often. The presence of protein and fats slows the absorption of carbohydrates, so, where it might be a bad idea to eat a pile of mashed potatoes alone, it's perfectly fine to eat modest servings in combination with a serving of meat and vegetables. For more information on this, see Nancy Appleton's classic book *Lick the Sugar Habit* (Avery 1996).

Keep most of your carb consumption in the low-GL section found at the top third of the chart. This gives your body the glucose it needs for fuel without the blood sugar spikes that leave you feeling tired and cranky and contribute to food cravings.

To further slow the glucose conversion, combine your carbs with protein. For example, add a couple of slices of roasted turkey to a piece of whole grain bread or have some poached salmon with a serving of brown rice.

What about low carb diets?

Low carb diets were all the rage a few years ago, then they were debunked because some researchers showed they might increase cholesterol and place undue strain on the liver.

However, many people had great success on these diets because they made weight control simple: Eat a lot of protein and few vegetables and a tiny amount of fruit and you'll lose weight.

Unfortunately, many people took the low carb-high protein concept as a license to chow down on bacon double cheeseburgers all day long. As long as we didn't eat the bun, it was great!

Not really.

Glycemic Index by Glycemic Load

	LOW GI*	MEDIUM GI	HIGH GI
LOW GL**	All-bran cereal (8, 42)	Beets (5, 64)	Popcorn (8, 72)
	Apples (6, 38)	Cantaloupe (4, 65)	Watermelon (4, 72)
	Carrots (3, 47)	Pineapple (7, 59)	Whole wheat flour bread (9, 71)
	Chana dal (3, 8)	Sucrose (table sugar) (7, 68)	White wheat flour bread (10, 70)
	Chickpeas (8, 28)		
	Grapes (8, 46)		
	Green peas (3, 48)		
	Kidney beans (7, 28)		
	Nopal (0, 7)		
	Oranges (5, 42)		
	Peaches (5, 42)		
	Peanuts (1, 14)		
	Pears (4, 38)		
	Pinto beans (10, 39)		
	Red lentils (5, 26)		
	Strawberries (1, 40)		
	Sweet corn (9, 54)		
MEDIUM GL	Apple juice (11, 40)	Life cereal (16, 66)	Cheerios (15, 74)
	Bananas (12, 52)	New potatoes (12, 57)	Shredded wheat (15, 75)
	Buckwheat (16, 54)	Sweet potatoes (17, 61)	
	Fettuccine (18, 40)	Wild rice (18, 57)	
	Navy beans (12, 38)		
	Orange juice (12, 50)		
	Parboiled rice (17, 47)		
	Pearled barley (11, 25)		
	Sourdough wheat bread (15, 54)		
HIGH GL	Linguine (23, 52)	Couscous (23, 65)	Baked russet potatoes (26, 85)
	Macaroni (23, 47)	White rice (23, 64)	Cornflakes (21, 81)
	Spaghetti (20, 42)		

*GI: low = 1–55, medium = 56–69, high = 70–100.

**GL: low = 1–10, medium = 11–19, high = 20 or more.

—Reprinted with permission: David Mendosa, www.mendosa.com, your online diabetes resource.

Recent research shows that a low carbohydrate/ high protein diet does result in more weight loss in the short term. It also can actually reduce the inflammatory markers that are signs of heart disease.

We recommend moderation. As part of a healthy eating plan, we need carbohydrates, but not in the quantities included in the SAD.

A moderately low carbohydrate diet is sensible if you use your daily carb allowance of 50 to 75 grams by eating whole grain cereals and breads and other complex carbohydrates that will give you long term energy.

The problem with the gimmicky diets that proclaim that carbohydrates will bring about the downfall of humankind is that you won't stick to them long. Above all, we prefer a healthy eating plan, not a diet.

Powered by Protein

The amount of protein you consume has a direct bearing on how you feel overall. Made up of amino acids, protein is the building block of all of the body's components, from hair and muscles to enzymes, hormones and neurotransmitters. Adequate protein intake can also boost your metabolism by 25%.

Our bodies require 23 different amino acids for proper function, 9 of them *essential*—lysine, tryptophane, methionine, valine, leucine, isoleucine, histidine, threonine and phenylalanine. Because our bodies cannot make them, they must be derived from our diet. We are able to manufacture the remaining amino acids, though at the cost of diverting precious materials and energy. So it's still better to eat as large a variety of amino acids as possible, even the so-called *nonessential* ones. The quality of a protein is determined by its balance of amino acids.

A complete protein is better absorbed and more efficiently utilized, so you will need a smaller amount of it to be optimally nourished. Meat, fish, chicken, poultry, cheese, milk and eggs are considered complete proteins because they contain the essential amino acids and in sufficient amounts.

We also prefer a diet that includes some meat, especially seafood and poultry because of their healthy fats and other nutrients.

However, if you choose a vegetarian diet, you can combine plant-based proteins that are missing one or two amino acids (e.g., soy is missing methionine) to create a complete protein. You can, for example, combine whole grains, nuts or seeds with a serving of beans or combine rice and beans for a complete protein.

You need about 20 grams of protein per meal. That is the equivalent of three eggs or three to four ounces of lean meat, poultry or fish or half a can (three ounces) of tuna.

Unpasteurized dairy products from a certified dairy that uses no antibiotics or hormones are also a good source of protein, provided you are not allergic to dairy. If you don't get unpasteurized, at least buy dairy products that are organic. Three small containers (16 ounces) of unsweetened yogurt or a cup of cottage cheese provide all you need. Soy hot dogs or burgers, five ounces of tofu or a serving of soy-based protein powder are good vegetarian options.

Whey-based protein powders are preferable to soy-based because whey is a more complete protein than soy and helps your body form the powerful antioxidant glutathione. There are hundreds of whey products on the market, so look for an organic, lactose-free (if you're lactose intolerant), sugar-free, low-carb whey protein product.

Vegetarians need to eat "seed" foods. These are foods that would grow if you planted them. These include seeds, nuts, beans, lentils, peas, corn, or the germ of grains such as wheat or oat. "Flower" foods, such as broccoli or cauliflower, are also relatively rich in protein. Lentils or beans plus brown rice provide an excellent source of complete protein.

A typical day might include a small container of yogurt and a heaping tablespoon of seeds on an oat-based cereal for breakfast and a 9.5-ounce serving of tofu and vegetable stir-fry served with either a cup of quinoa or a serving of beans with rice as part of dinner.

Other choices include eating a peanut butter sandwich or tossing almonds or walnuts into a whole grain pasta recipe.

VEGETABLE PROTEIN CHOICES

Grains/Legumes: tofu, lentils, chickpeas, quinoa, millet, brown rice

Nuts/Seeds: pumpkin seeds, sunflower seeds, almonds, cashew nuts, walnuts

Vegetables: broccoli, spinach, peas, beans

Combinations: lentils and rice, beans and rice

Fats are Essential

Most of us realize by now that fats don't make you fat. In fact, certain fats are essential to keep your body healthy. The low-fat diet craze of the past 20 years has led to a nationwide epidemic of obesity and can cause everything from PMS and infertility to depression, anxiety and even premature aging. The strongest supporting evidence that the low-fat boom led to the current obesity trend lies in the numbers.

According to the Center for Health Statistics, the American obesity epidemic started in the early 1980s. Not coincidentally at the same time, the market was flooded with low-fat products. Suddenly, the rate of overweight adults went through the roof, nearly skyrocketing from a steady 13 to 14% at the beginning of the '80s to a rate approaching 25% by the end of the decade and now encompassing more than one-third of all Americans.

Fats are important, too.

High quality fats are an essential part of human life. We need them for all body functions ranging from heart health and energy metabolism to brain function. The best sources of these healthy fats are cold water fish like salmon and tuna and oils made from nuts and seeds.

About 30% of the calories in your diet should come from good fats. The best fats are healthy polyunsaturated fatty acids such as fish oil, flaxseed oil, and borage oil. These are omega-3 and omega-6 fatty acids that stimulate the immune system and fight inflammation that can cause heart disease and many other chronic diseases. They also support optimal brain function.

Omega-3s are found in fish, especially in fatty fish like salmon, tuna and mackerel and in flaxseeds (though in a less usable form). The omega-6 fatty acids are found in meat, milk, vegetable oils, seeds and nuts. Most of us consume too many omega-6 fatty acids, even though minimal quantities are good for us.

For an adequate omega-3 supply, you should eat fatty fish three times a week or take 1,000–2,000 mg of fish oil daily as a supplement according to label instructions. Note: Be careful of eating too much fish. Even wild caught fish have recently found to have potentially dangerous mercury levels.

You can add good fats by sprinkling a heaping tablespoon of ground flaxseed on salads, cereals or vegetables every day.

Organic cold-pressed seed oil blends like flaxseed, soybean, sesame, walnut and almond provide the right fats with omega-6 and omega-3 fatty acids in a ratio of approximately 3:1. Most of us eat about 20 times more omega-6 fatty acids than omega-3s in products like cereals, whole grain bread, baked goods, fried foods, margarine and others.

It's important to used cold-pressed oils because the heat and chemicals used in other types of refining processes destroy the essential fatty acids (EFA). You can't cook with most cold-pressed oils because they degrade when heated. Use them on salads, put them on baked potatoes in place of butter and drizzle them over steamed veggies for a delicious treat.

Olive oil and cold-pressed sesame oil can be used for cooking at low temperatures, but you may lose some of the healthiest ingredients if you attempt to use them to fry foods. Better yet, give up fried foods.

- Reduce your intake of beef and pork because they are high in saturated fat, a less healthy form of fat, which is also likely to contain hormones, antibiotics and pesticide residues. Organic meats and grass-fed cattle to reduce the hazards of chemicals and hormones considerably. They also give you a good source of CLA (conjugated linoleic acid), which has been shown to be helpful in weight control. Eat the leanest cuts possible.

- Skinless chicken and turkey (also organic, if possible) are better sources of proteins, without too much saturated fat. Eggs contain omega-3 fatty acids as well, with the docosahexanoic acid (DHA)–enriched eggs from organically raised chickens containing 200 mg of omega-3 fatty acids in each egg.

- Completely eliminate trans-fatty acids from your diet. Become a label reader, and avoid anything that says it contains hydrogenated or partially hydrogenated vegetable oils. Those are just benign-sounding names for artery-clogging trans fatty acids. Trans-fatty acids are found in most baked goods and many processed foods. Buyer beware: Most fast-food is drenched in trans fats and French fries are the worst culprit.

Phospholipids

We are fatheads! Our brain cells are made up of 60% fats or lipids, primarily the phospholipids phosphatidylcholine and phosphatidylserine. They form the insulating layer, or myelin sheath, that covers all nerve cells. They enhance circulation, liver function and mental performance, protecting against age-related memory decline and Alzheimer's disease.

Although your body can make them, getting extra phospholipids from food is highly beneficial. Egg yolk is the richest source of phospholipids in the average diet. However, ever since egg phobia set in as part of the cholesterol scare, the average intake of phospholipids has dropped dramatically. The American Heart Association now states that you can eat up to seven eggs a week without negatively affecting your cholesterol.

Significantly, since we as a society became egg-phobic, cases of Alzheimer's disease have skyrocketed.

Lecithin is an excellent source of phospholipids and is widely available in health food stores as either granules or capsules. The easiest and cheapest way to add lecithin to your diet is to sprinkle a tablespoon of lecithin granules or a heaping teaspoon of high-PC lecithin on your cereal or add it to your protein drink in the morning. Or you can take four lecithin capsules providing 1,200 mg each. By the way, lecithin doesn't make you fat. In fact, quite the opposite occurs: It helps your body to break down fat.

EAT YOUR FRUITS AND VEGETABLES

Eat at least five servings a day of fruits and vegetables. The beneficial plant chemicals or phytonutrients come in a great variety of colors. Although there are 150,000 edible plant species on earth, most people limit themselves to iceberg lettuce, tomatoes, potatoes (including French fries), bananas, and oranges (mainly as juice).

Studies have shown repeatedly that fruits and veggies protect us against many diseases including cancer, stroke and degenerative diseases.

Think of a rainbow of colors, fresh and unusual! Picture a cornucopia of fruits and vegetables: crunchy orange carrots, deep purple eggplants, bright red plump tomatoes, shiny green peppers, luscious purple grapes, abundant green leaves of lettuce, kale, and spinach, yellow and green squash, and large juicy peaches. These are Nature's gifts, filled with an incredible array of vitamins, minerals and phytonutrients that nourish and heal us. The deeper the color, the more antioxidants and other beneficial phytochemicals you're getting. They have fiber that aids in digestion and sugars that break down slowly for steady energy, and some even have some protein.

Buy your fruits and vegetables fresh as much as you can. The highest nutritional values are found in fruits and vegetables grown close to home, vine-ripened and harvested shortly before they land on your table.

Next best is frozen.

The worst choice, in most cases, is canned foods because the heat processing has cooked most of the nutrients out of the plant. The exception to the canned rule: tomatoes and beans. The nutritional values of tomatoes and beans are actually enhanced by the canning process.

You can eat vegetables raw, steamed or lightly sautéed in olive oil. The varieties are endless. Eat all different colors for the different chemicals, each with its own special benefits. Add healthy salad dressings, ones without sugar, MSG and other chemicals. Or make your own with sesame oil, soy sauce and some spices and herbs that have their own nutritional value.

Microwaving vegetables is a poor choice since the microwaving process robs foods of most of their nutrients.

SPICES AND HERBS

Besides taste, herbs and seasonings provide missing elements in the diet. Here are just a few of the herbal superstars of the kitchen that have known healing effects: cinnamon, cilantro, parsley, garlic, oregano, turmeric (cumin), ginger and rosemary.

The Salt Issue

Limit your intake of normal table salt. It is processed sodium chloride and is as bad for you as any other processed food. On the other hand, sea salt in its natural form is essential for good cellular function. It contains all the minerals, including iodine, and trace minerals in the correct ratio relative to blood plasma. Salt is particularly important for pituitary, thyroid, adrenal, kidney and pancreas function. In fact, many of the people who crave salt have low thyroid and adrenal function and are seeking balance. Rather than reaching for the potato chips, though, add pure sea or other unprocessed salt to your food, in moderation.

ANTIOXIDANTS

Oxygen is the ultimate "essential." A few minutes without it and you're dead. We use it to help burn our food to produce energy. The trouble is, whenever we make energy, we also produce toxic by-products called free radicals. One puff of a cigarette, for example, lets loose a trillion free radical molecules in the smoker. Exhaust fumes, pollution, fried and browned foods and exposure to the sun can be equally disastrous. Free radicals are the major cause of the aging process. They attack brain cells and are largely responsible for the decline in the number of brain cells as we age.

How can you keep free radicals at bay? Increase your intake of antioxidants, a family of nutrients with the power to mop them up and so reverse the aging process. Top antioxidants include prunes, raisins, pomegranates, blueberries and blackberries. Kale, spinach, strawberries, raspberries, plums, broccoli and alfalfa sprouts are nearly as powerful.

Make sure your daily supplement program contains significant quantities of antioxidants, especially if you live in a polluted city or have any other unavoidable exposure.

A comprehensive antioxidant supplement, together with a good multivitamin and mineral tablet, is the best way to go. Each works in its own way, and they work together synergistically. Most high-quality supplement companies produce combination formulas with the following nutrients: vitamin A, beta-carotene, vitamin E, vitamin C, zinc, selenium, glutathione and cysteine, plus plant-based antioxidants such as anthocyanidins from a source such as bilberry or pycnogenol. For more on toxins and antioxidants, see Chapters 6 and 15.

ADD MULTIVITAMINS

To achieve optimum health and nutrition, you need to "eat right *and* take a multivitamin," as a recent headline in a *New England Journal of Medicine* editorial put it. "The evidence suggests that people who take such supplements and their children are healthier."

Vitamins and minerals function as cofactors, or chemical helpers, in the chemical processes that are occurring at every moment in each and every cell of your body. For instance, B vitamins can protect you from depression, anxiety, stress, confusion, fatigue, mental dullness, and emotional fragility, and can even boost IQ.

The minerals magnesium (Mg), iron (Fe), zinc (Zn), manganese (Mn) and chromium (Cr), plus antioxidant nutrients, especially vitamin C, are also vital for brain power and overall health. Other benefits include enhanced energy, memory, blood sugar regulation and immunity.

Although the recommended daily intake (RDI) of essential nutrients is intended to be available entirely through food, in reality, it is impossible to get these levels through the food available to us today because our soil has become depleted in essential nutrients, so the fresh and wholesome foods that are being grown have lower quantities of these essential vitamins and minerals than they had 50 or 100 years ago. Add to this the loss of nutrients in transit from farm to table.

Recent analyses of nearly a dozen popular diet plans show that none of them provide 100% of the RDAs (the government's Recommended Daily Intakes) for 13 vitamins and minerals. Finally, the RDAs are a one-size-fits-all approach to nutrition, and each of us is different. Individual physiology, lifestyle, stress, age and physical condition all weigh heavily on our nutritional needs. And the RDA really is not enough to keep us in optimal health.

Consider this research. Ninety students were assigned to one of three groups: one received a multivitamin and mineral supplement; the second received an identical-looking placebo; and the third, nothing. After seven months, the IQs of those taking the supplements had increased by a staggering nine points! A five-point increase would get half the learning-disabled children out of special schools and back to normal schooling.

My pet project, Nourish America, which supplies at-risk children around the country with daily multivitamin/mineral tablets has shown similar results: better health, less absenteeism and aggression and improved learning and behavior.

Nourish America has also supplied vitamins to seniors who are at risk of malnutrition, and we have received wonderful letters, thanking us for the difference our vitamins have made in their health and well-being. Learn more at www.nourishamerica.org.

If you're not already taking a high-potency multivitamin, start taking one now that contains the approximate amounts of the essential vitamins and minerals shown in Optimal Supplement Program below

Doses may vary in different formulas. Food-based formulas, for example, are likely to have lower but not necessarily less-potent doses.

You will probably need to take anywhere from four to six capsules a day to provide all the necessary ingredients. Capsules are generally preferable to tablets because they have with fewer additives and fillers, and are easier to digest and absorb.

Your multi-vitamin formula should use natural ingredients, meaning they are purely natural and not synthetic and that contain no unnatural ingredients such as preservatives, sugar, tar, artificial color or flavoring

Start with one or two daily and gradually work your way up to the recommended dose. Take them with food both to aid in their digestion and to prevent side effects such as the nausea that affects some women, often due to the B vitamins.

Calcium and magnesium are quite bulky, at nearly 2,000 mg for the combination and aren't always included in sufficient quantities in a multi vitamin, so be sure to add them in if your supplement contains less than 1,000 mg of calcium and 400 mg of magnesium.

You also need 1,000 to 2,000 mg of vitamin C daily, and more if you are coming down with a cold or have an infection of any kind.

Take at least, 1,000 mg of essential fatty acids daily, preferably in the form of fish oil rather than flax oil, because fish oil contains both of the essential fatty acids, EPA (eicosopentanoic acid) and DHA (docosahexanoic acid). Although our bodies are supposed to be able to convert EPA to DHA, not everyone can do it efficiently. In this case, the fish has already done it for us!

There is plenty of evidence for the benefits of fish oil in a variety of conditions, including cardiovascular disease, hormonal imbalance, bipolar illness, depression, alcoholism, and postpartum depression. A vegetarian alternative is to also combine flax oil with algae-based sources of DHA.

Take at least 30 mg of coenzyme Q_{10}, more if you can. You can go up to 1 mg per pound of body weight and those quantities are not generally included in a multivitamin.

ADD PROBIOTICS

Probiotics, literally meaning "for life," are the friendly bacteria that reside in our digestive tracts. They help us to digest our food and absorb its nutrients, manufacture vitamins B, A, and K and maintain optimal immune function. In short, they promote good health. Unfortunately, these natural intestinal flora are often destroyed by antibiotics, birth control pills, stress, alcohol, acid-blocking drugs and infections.

The easiest way to include probiotics in your diet is to add a cup of organic yogurt to your food plan every day, one that says it contains live, active cultures. However, because the probiotic content of manufactured yogurt is not always reliable, it is still better to take probiotics in capsules, tablets, beverages, and powders, which are available at health food stores everywhere.

Take a six-week course of these healthy bacteria to restore your normal gut flora, and longer if you have chronic intestinal problems (Chapter 14). Look for a product supplying five billion bacteria—including *Lactobacillus acidophilus* and *Bifidobacterium*—per day in divided doses (twice daily before meals). Enteric-coated products are preferred because they protect the bacteria from being destroyed by stomach acid en route to the intestines, where they do their work. Lactobacilli are sensitive to light, heat and moisture, so use refrigerated products in an opaque, moisture-proof container. There are products on the market that don't need refrigeration, as well.

CLEAN OUT YOUR PANTRY

This week, go through the food in your house. Become a label reader. A simple rule of thumb: if you can't pronounce it, don't eat it! Our food supply is loaded with chemicals and we're fortunate that some (not all) of them are listed on food labels. The purpose of most of those chemicals is to preserve food. Because you're moving toward a diet rich in whole, fresh, and healthy foods, these nonfoods have no place in your life.

Get rid of the sugar and the nutritionally depleted white flour and white rice. Most cereal, cookies, and baked goods are packed with sugar and harmful fats. Into the trash bin they go. Ditto for zero-nutrient, sugared (or chemically sweetened), caffeinated soft drinks. This covers virtually all soft drinks, diet or not.

Canned fruits and vegetables (with the exception of tomatoes and beans) are usually so overprocessed that all vitamins are cooked right out of them. We recommend fresh or frozen fruits and vegetables.

You can keep organic, whole grain foods and cereals.

Certainly you should toss out solid shortenings like Crisco and boxed mixes like (yuck!) Hamburger Helper.

Finally, if you have decided to go on the Vibrant Health Plan, it may be difficult to drag your family kicking and screaming along with you. Be a bit flexible, especially if your family is accustomed to a diet high in sugary and processed foods. Introduce the new regimen gradually and you'll probably have little resistance. After all, you are following basic food truths that will benefit anyone's health.

At the market, shop the perimeter where the produce is and buy organic whenever possible.

VIBRANT HEALTH BASICS

• Make sure most of your diet is made up of whole foods and fresh foods.

• Eat three servings a day of top-quality proteins like fish, organic poultry or lean meat, egg (free range), soy or combinations of beans, lentils and grains.

• Avoid hydrogenated fats, and reduce your intake of saturated fats from meat, dairy and junk food.

• Choose low-GL carbohydrates such as whole grains, vegetables, and most fruits and avoid sugar and refined foods.

• Eat fish three times a week or take fish oil supplements.

• Use cold-pressed seed oils in salad dressings.

• Drink at least two quarts of water a day, either pure or in diluted juices and herbal or fruit teas.

• Minimize your intake of tea, coffee and alcohol.

• Eat at least five servings a day of antioxidant-rich fruits and vegetables.

• Take these supplements daily: a high-potency multivitamin and mineral formula, 1–3 g of vitamin C, an antioxidant formula, and 1,000–2,000 mg of essential fatty acids.

6

WEEK 6

Detoxify Your Body

———

Continue with your nutrition, supplement, and exercise routines, as you will do throughout your entire Vibrant Health Plan.

Now we'll address the toxins in our bodies. Sad to say, we are living in a sea of poisons. We hear the stories on the news every day. Even the polar bears in the Arctic are loaded with mercury from eating mercury-laden fish. Inuit children have pesticides in their bloodstreams carried by air and sea and through the food they eat.

Newborn babies are shown to have high levels of chemicals in their systems. In 2004, researchers found a total of 287 industrial chemicals and pollutants in umbilical cord blood, including pesticides, consumer product ingredients and wastes from burning coal, gasoline and garbage in the blood of newborns. We know that 180 of these toxins cause cancer in humans or animals, 217 are toxic to the brain and nervous system and 208 cause birth defects or abnormal development in animal tests. These clearly pose a serious threat to the growth, development and overall health of these children.

The average American consumes about 14 pounds of chemicals a year in the form of food additives such as artificial food coloring, flavorings, emulsifiers, humectants, and preservatives. Then, beyond the known "bad stuff" that we ingest more or less voluntarily, we are also exposed to environmental toxins caused by everything from contaminated food to air pollution and secondhand cigarette smoke.

There are industrial wastes, hydrocarbons, chemical fertilizers, and pesticides in our air, water and food supplies. And don't forget the hormones and antibiotics that pollute most of our meat and dairy products.

Even generally healthy foods like fish can be a source of toxic mercury and long-term exposure to heavy metals can cause brain and nervous system damage.

All of us are exposed to some or even many of these toxins. Most of us are not sick because of them, but it's a fine line between "OK" and "toxin overload." Toxins build up in our bodies, and we may not even notice their effects for years until the load becomes too great, we become imbalanced and the scales tip, causing a wide range of health problems, including headaches, fatigue, muscle weakness and more.

Because toxins are unavoidable, we're recommending a simple detoxification process here. If toxin imbalance is a major factor in your symptoms, you'll want to explore these issues more deeply with the recommendations in Chapter 15.

In addition to these chemical poisons, many women have food allergies or, more properly, food sensitivities, some of which they're not even aware of. For details, see Chapter 14.

Here's a basic detox diet:

For the next week, avoid or drastically reduce your intake of the following:

- Refined sugars

- Alcohol

- Caffeine

- Wheat and other gluten products (barley, rye, oats)

- Dairy products

- Corn and all corn products, especially high-fructose corn syrup

- Canned and processed foods

- Food additives, preservatives, and artificial flavorings

- Hydrogenated and partially hydrogenated vegetable oils, including margarine, shortening, and most commercial salad dressings and sauces

You can eat the following:

- Animal protein: Skinless organic poultry, eggs and wild game
- Wild caught cold water fish: Not more than two servings a week
- Tofu and tempeh
- Organic sheep and goat's milk products, organic yogurt, and organic butter
- Rice, millet, quinoa
- Vegetables (all except corn), organic if possible
- All dried beans and legumes
- Fruit (organic, if possible), fresh or frozen
- Extra-virgin cold-pressed olive oil, sesame, or macadamia nut oil for cooking
- Flaxseed oil for dressings
- Bottled spring water, which contains minerals not present in filtered water
- Fruit juices (diluted 50% or more with water), vegetable juices, herbal teas, rice milk

This diet will bring you back to simplicity in your eating patterns. It is not intended as a weight-loss diet, but you are likely to lose some weight. What will happen is that you will begin to clear your system of toxins and food allergies.

You'll likely notice an improvement in your energy levels and other symptoms as the week goes on. You will also be introduced (or reintroduced) to the taste of real, fresh, whole food, just as nature made it. Whether they are steamed, raw, braised, you will find a new delight in these simple foods.

If you experience flu-like symptoms in the first few days, don't give up! Among your toxins may be yeasts and parasites. When they are deprived of the sugars that feed them, they begin to die, releasing their toxins into your system and causing temporary discomfort called "die-off." If this happens, drink more water, add 1,000 to 2,000 mg more vitamin C as a supplement, and read Chapter 14, where you'll find a more rigorous detox program to overcome intestinal yeast problems. On the other hand, there is a good chance that this detox alone will take care of your problem.

If you want to increase the power of this simple cleanse, follow the recommendations in Ann-Louise Gittleman's book *The Fat Flush Plan* (McGraw-Hill, 2002). It's an excellent book, with clear explanations and guidelines. One of Gittleman's most helpful suggestions is to drink eight glasses of unsweetened cranberry juice diluted with water. The easiest way to do this is to put 4 ounces of cranberry juice in a 32-ounce bottle and fill the bottle with water. You'll need two bottles of the juice cocktail a day.

To add even more power to the cleanse, take 100 mg of the herb *milk thistle* (also called silymarin) twice a day to help support your liver in the detoxification efforts.

An important point here is to be sure you are having regular bowel movements. Yup, we do have to cover this often-avoided topic. Many toxins are released into the bowel, so if it's not moving, neither are these poisons.

Believe it or not, you should be having one to two bowel movements a day, each about two feet long and about the diameter of a 50 cent piece. I bet no one ever told you that one! It should float and break apart when you flush. Otherwise, you are missing essential fatty acids, friendly bacteria, or fiber.

In addition to the fiber from fruits and vegetables, you can add a teaspoon of psyllium husks to your cranberry juice, once or twice daily, first thing in the morning or in the evening, between dinner and bedtime. And continue with a minimum of eight glasses of water (or cranberry cocktail). The bottom line here is once you remove the toxic energy robbers from your life, you will have far more vitality.

Be sure to fill in your journal, especially the food-mood-supplement-activity record. You will be able to look back and track your "good" and "bad" foods.

STARTING BACK

The next step will be gradually introducing certain foods back into your diet one at a time to tell what effect they are having on you.

Challenge You may be feeling much better after the elimination phase of your eating plan. You'll start experimenting by eating a portion of a suspect food. For example, if you think you have a problem with dairy products, drink a glass or two of milk and record your state at intervals over the next couple of days. Only challenge with one food at a time and space your challenges by at least 24 hours, preferably more so there is no confusion about which food you are tracking. This takes into account the "delayed sensitivity" that characterizes many food allergies. This will probably take several weeks, but you'll be developing a list of your hidden food allergies that will serve you well.

Reassessment. If you're still having symptoms, you'll need to dig deeper into the sources of your food sensitivities. Progressively eliminate some of the basic foods that were allowed during the elimination phase and see if you get results.

Maintenance. Now that you've discovered your triggers, you can lighten up a bit on the program. You can fine-tune your personal program because you know what works. If you challenged yourself on a food and passed the test, add moderate amounts back into your diet, but probably not more than three or four times per week. Called *rotation,* this spacing of potential allergens makes them less likely to become problematic in the future.

Again, your journal should be stuck to you: record all your reactions. Don't waste a minute of this precious opportunity to learn about your food reactions.

BREAKING YOUR ADDICTIONS

If you cringe at the thought of stopping sugar, alcohol, and caffeine or if you're a smoker, turn to this section before doing the detox. It will help you to understand the issues of addiction and its relationship to brain chemistry. You can then modify the detox to accommodate your imbalanced brain chemistry. You can still do the diet, but add in the suggested supplements to help with the cravings.

Do you crave that first morning cup of coffee or really look forward to your coffee break?

- Do you find you can't wait to get home for your after-work drink and can't relax without it?

- Do you prefer dessert to dinner?

- Are you secretive about how much you smoke?

You're not alone. Here's a story that may seem familiar, if not to you, then to someone you know.

Margo, a 35-year-old flight attendant, came to see me for a "tune-up." She noticed she was more tired and less able to adapt to time zone changes than in the past. When asked to describe her diet, she was quick to warn, "Don't make me give up my drink before dinner!"

It was Margo's attachment to her drink that was the clue to how dependent she was on it. If alcohol held no charge for Margo, she wouldn't have even thought of mentioning it. We're not talking about the one drink a day. We're talking about the attitude. Substitute any other addiction and you'll see what we mean: the late-afternoon candy bar, the eagerly anticipated cigarette break or the morning coffee.

When women like Margo have problems with a substance, it's usually not that they are weak-willed or have an "addictive personality." They simply have an underlying chemical imbalance that is depleting their energy and peace of mind and they don't even know it. For details, see Chapter 10 on how your brain chemistry "makes you do it," as well as Chapters 12 and 13.

Whether it's sugar, caffeine, alcohol, soft drinks or tobacco, your dependence on them undermines your health. I seldom tell my patients that they "have to" stop or even reduce these addictive substances. The secret is that once you are on a well-balanced and nutritious diet and taking the right supplements, the cravings disappear! That's because they are symptoms of an imbalance that, once corrected, frees you of the compulsion. You are then able to *choose* a drink with dinner or a cookie for dessert (and not a whole box of them, a sign of sugar addiction). Or not. There is no inner conflict involved here.

When diet alone doesn't work, research shows we can successfully treat addiction and cravings with the use of specific amino acids. These include the precursors (building blocks) of the neurotransmitters serotonin, dopamine, glutamine, and GABA (gamma-aminobutyric acid, which is both a neurotransmitter and an amino acid) (see Chapter 10).

When neurotransmitter precursors were given to alcoholic subjects, the individuals experienced fewer cravings for alcohol, less stress, increased likelihood of recovery, and fewer relapses.

You'll notice no mention of the word *willpower*. It is clear that most addictions are the result of chemical imbalances based on your genes, your diet and your lifestyle and are not that hard to correct if approached in this manner.

If you have cravings for fast food, doughnuts and high-sugar foods, coffee, tea, soft drinks, chocolate, alcohol or any other substance, we have a simple answer for you—see the "Quick Tip to Stop Cravings."

QUICK TIP TO STOP CRAVINGS

Keep a bottle of 500 mg capsules of L-glutamine on hand. This amino acid can cut a craving almost on the spot. When a craving strikes, take a 500 mg capsule, open it up, and pour the contents directly under your tongue. It's absorbed quickly and will give you an almost instant pick-me-up similar to your longed-for stimulant, alcohol included. You can also take glutamine several times a day, between meals, to prevent cravings. Add 500 mg of D,L-phenylalanine or tyrosine two to three times a day, and your energy will be high and stay that way, with no more cravings!

REDUCE SUGAR

Refined sugar adds calories and has no food value. What's more, high-sugar foods like soft drinks, doughnuts and candy lead to a mood roller coaster called the "sugar blues." First these foods cause a rapid rise in blood sugar (glucose), requiring your body to secrete more insulin to cope with it. The insulin then removes this excess sugar from the blood and stores it as fat and glycogen. This causes your blood sugar levels to drop and making you feel weak, light-headed, and even cranky. See more details on this in Chapter 13.

What about sugar substitutes? Diet drinks contain the artificial sweetener aspartame (brand names NutraSweet, Equal), which can be toxically overstimulating to the brain. I've seen patients who thought they were going crazy with jitters, insomnia and disordered thinking, who magically recovered when they stopped drinking diet sodas! Ironically, although touted as a diet product, these drinks can actually cause weight gain. When consumed with carbohydrates, aspartame inhibits the production of a brain chemical that signals fullness. See www.dorway.com/blayenn.html for scientific information on aspartame.

To get over an aspartame addiction, try the amino acid D,L-phenylalanine.

The jury is still out on Splenda®, which is produced by chlorinating sugar (sucrose). There have been no long-term human studies on its use and no independent monitoring of health effects.

Since we don't really know how safe Splenda is, it's best to err on the side of caution. A little once in a while probably isn't a big problem, but keep your consumption to a minimum.

Eliminating sugar- and caffeine-containing soft drinks will move you strongly in the right direction.

To take care of those other cravings, you can substitute a 2-ounce pack of raw (and preferably unsalted) nuts for your afternoon candy bar and you won't get sugar withdrawal. In fact, you'll probably experience quite the opposite. You'll notice the difference in your energy levels right away. Most kinds of nuts are excellent sources of healthy fats. Almonds, cashews, and walnuts are particularly good sources of protein as well.

If you really like your sweets, try xylitol, an excellent sugar substitute that has health benefits as well: it helps to prevent tooth decay by preventing the growth of bacteria in the mouth. Another good choice is stevia, a supersweet herbal extract that may even help lower blood sugar. Stevia is easily found at health food stores in both liquid and powdered form. It works best in drinks. It doesn't work as well in baking because heating changes the flavor.

The addition of complex carbohydrates, including more high-fiber foods, will go a long way toward allaying your sugar cravings. Add some protein and a dose of chromium (200 mcg), and you are far less likely to go on a sugar binge.

For alcohol cravings, balance your sugar and add 500 mg of glutamine daily. This little step has miraculously turned around a number of my heavy-drinking patients relatively painlessly.

An excellent book that discusses emotional reasons as well as physiological reasons for food cravings is Nan Fuchs' *Overcoming the Legacy of Overeating: How to Change Your Negative Eating Patterns* (McGraw-Hill, 1999) for which I wrote the foreword.

REDUCE CAFFEINE

If you're a coffee or soft drink junkie, now is the time to start gradually cutting back. If you're heavily into caffeine, stopping cold turkey might give you withdrawal headaches. This happens because your blood vessels have been accustomed to being constricted from the caffeine. As they dilate to a normal level, the increased circulation is experienced as a headache. You'll be fine with a gradual reduction; the goal is to eliminate caffeine entirely, because it creates a stress response and can give you the jitters. Even that one cup in the morning can disrupt sleep patterns, as well. Caffeine may also raise blood pressure, blood sugar, and cholesterol and contributes to breast lumps called fibrocystic breasts. Reduce your caffeine input by one-third this week, reduce it by another one-third next week, and cut it out completely by the third week.

Shifting to green tea is an option. While containing caffeine, it also contains healthy substances that can lower cholesterol and blood pressure, enhance immune function and speed up metabolism and weight loss. One or two cups daily, not close to bedtime, should not be a problem.

Yerba mate is another low-caffeine substitute with many health benefits, and it is available at health food stores (see www.guayaki.com for lots of good information on this South American herb). Another option is Teeccino, a delicious, herbal, caffeine-free substitute that is prepared just like coffee and is available in health food stores (www.teecino.com).

D,L-phenylalanine and tyrosine, 500 mg can help you deal with caffeine cravings. You can preempt the need for both your wake-up coffee and your midmorning cup with a capsule or two of one of these stimulating amino acids without the negative effects of coffee. Once you are over your cravings, you may be able to drop these amino acids, using them only as needed.

STOP SMOKING

We realize that smoking is an extremely difficult habit to overcome. Yet it is the single most hazardous thing you can do to your health.

In 2005, more than 79,000 women in the United States died from lung cancer. That is more than the number of women died from breast, ovarian, and uterine cancers combined. Cigarette smoking is the primary cause of lung cancer, and approximately 22 million women in the United States smoke. Between 1930 and 1997, the number of lung cancer deaths in women in the United States has increased by 600%. Most of the deaths can be attributed to an increase in cigarette smoking by women.

Smoking can relax you, curb your appetite and give you a lift. All of this is due to nicotine's action on brain chemistry, blood sugar and adrenal hormones. Your purified diet and supplementation program may actually reduce your cravings.

Start paying attention to your smoking habits. These habits, or any habits, can be triggered by a specific situation, like Pavlov's dog trained to salivate at the sound of the bell right before he was fed. Make a list of those triggers and then change the habit. If you habitually smoke after meals, get up and do something else the moment you're finished eating. If you smoke when you're upset, try listening to your favorite music or taking a walk instead. If you usually smoke after sex, either stop having sex (just kidding!) or find a healthier alternative to its aftermath. After you've eliminated the habitual "smoking times," you'll find your urges to smoke have been vastly reduced.

TIPS TO QUITTING SMOKING

1. Resist the urges to substitute sugar, fatty food, alcohol or other stimulants for nicotine. In fact, your efforts to cut out sugar and other stimulants from your diet will pay off big time in getting the nicotine monkey off your back because the craving cycle has already been interrupted.

2. Eat small, frequent meals with lots of slow-releasing complex carbohydrates combined with protein-rich foods.

3. Reduce your nicotine load by gradually switching to brands with less nicotine until the brand you smoke has no more than 2 mg of nicotine per cigarette.

4. Be sure you're getting the following supplements every day, in addition to your multivitamin:
   - Vitamin C: at least 1,000 mg to cut cravings and help flush nicotine out of your system
   - Chromium: 100 mcg to balance blood sugars and eliminate cravings
   - Niacin: 50 mg to neutralize the nicotine's effects (Note: you may experience a hot, prickly rash spreading from your face down about 15 to 30 minutes after you take niacin. This will disappear after about 15 minutes. Taking it with food reduces this effect. It also diminishes with subsequent doses. If the flush is too uncomfortable (some women like it), you could substitute nonflush niacin inositol hexanicotinate.
   - Calcium-magnesium, 1:1 ratio: 500 mg each, above what you are already taking. Both calcium and magnesium are alkaline minerals that will help to neutralize the acidity that leads to cravings.
   - Lecithin: 2 tablespoons of granules dissolved in juice or water to reduce cravings
   - 5-HTP (5-hydroxytryptophan): 100 mg twice a day or 200 mg an hour before bed to help raise serotonin levels, banishing depression and irritability caused by nicotine withdrawal
   - DLPA or tyrosine: 500–1,000 mg, one to two times daily to replace the pickup that you're used to getting from nicotine

Nicotine affects adrenal hormones, blood sugar, and brain chemicals, so stabilizing adrenal function (Chapter 12), blood sugar (Chapter 13), hormone levels (Chapter 11) and your brain chemistry (Chapter 10) will help diminish your tobacco cravings as well.

Margo did the detox plan and learned a great deal about herself. When she had been off sugar for a week and then added some to her herbal tea, she became wired. About an hour later, she felt very sleepy. She was still quite burned out at that stage and her adrenals had little reserve, giving her that exaggerated response. These reactions had been occurring all along but had been "masked" by her long-term sugar habit. That's why it's a good idea to stop potential problem foods and then watch your response when they are reintroduced, one at a time.

Margo didn't even want to test herself on alcohol. Had she not been taking supplements, I would also have been concerned about her going off the wagon. No problem here. In fact, her obligatory daily wine craving ended quite easily. As her nutritional status improved with a good diet, multivitamins and amino acids, she forgot her habit. The last opened bottle of wine actually sat in the refrigerator until her roommate finally used it for cooking!

NAET DESENSITIZATION

Many practitioners use a simple desensitization technique called Nambudripad's Allergy Elimination Technique (NAET), named for the southern California doctor who developed it. It uses a diagnostic technique in which an indicator muscle is used to determine if a particular substance causes a weakness in the person's energy field, as reflected by the muscle strength.

Acupuncture or acupressure is then used to treat the weakness. The patient can often resume eating the offending food or be exposed to the chemical without further problems. While this sounds unlikely, the results are compelling. It helps to remember that Westerners were very skeptical of acupuncture itself when they first heard of it. If you are interested in NAET, look for a practitioner at www.naet.com. I have applied it to help stop sugar and alcohol cravings, as well. While it's not 100% effective, it continues to be helpful in dealing with food allergies and cravings.

7

WEEK 7

Exercise and Self-Care

You've identified the most likely underlying causes of your health problems, read the pertinent chapters, and made some positive changes. This week's focus is on external factors that can help bring you back to vibrant health. We want you to look and feel your best, and this week's Vibrant Health Plan is going to give you some exciting tools to help you get there.

A healthy woman exudes an aura of vibrancy and well-being. Just think about a woman you know who has that special something that makes her attractive far beyond her physical beauty. Chances are she's in the peak of physical condition, regardless of her chronological age. That kind of health expresses itself in clear skin and eyes, healthy hair, good posture and a relaxed and easy grace that's difficult to describe.

The secret to this kind of glowing health lies in exercise, stress management and skin and hair care. Think of this week as your spa week, the week your body and spirit begin to take on that glow.

EXERCISE

Let's face it: Most of us don't get enough exercise. We all have dozens of reasons, and we all have busy schedules. The truth is that it is difficult for many of us to find time to fit exercise into our lives.

Setting aside your personal time every day, especially your exercise time, will actually give you more time for the rest of your activities. Exercise energizes, focuses and tones every cell in your body, not just your muscles.

That means your daily workout will give you more energy, more mental clarity and less stress, making your day run more smoothly. You'll actually find you get more done if you spend that half hour working out in the morning, take a brisk walk at lunchtime or attend a Pilates class after work.

What works? There are hundreds of exercise methods, so the best one is what works for you. The key to a successful program is to choose an approach to exercise that you truly enjoy.

A failed exerciser is invariably the one who joined a hard-body workout class just because a neighbor invited her or went for a yoga class when she really wanted to run a couple of miles on the beach. What's right for you won't necessarily be right for your neighbor or even your best friend.

You make the choice. It's not important what form of exercise you choose, but that you stay with a program. And you'll stay with a program you love. It's as simple as that. We promise you'll be happier and healthier in the long run.

Give some thought to these questions:

- Are you very social and love to be around lots of people? If so, joining a gym, a hiking club or an aerobics class may be the answer for you.

- Or do you love individual challenges and think the best competition is against your own personal best? Think about speed walking, running or mountain biking.

- Or are you the quiet type who loves solitude and sees exercise time as a time of reflection and quiet contemplation? Your answer might lie in hiking, yoga, swimming or working out in a home gym.

Once you've decided what type of exerciser you're likely to be, we're going to shake up your world a little by telling you that the best exercise is varied. Don't do the same thing every day. It's bound to become boring! Studies also show that variety pushes your body to work harder: As your body becomes accustomed to an exercise, it actually becomes more efficient at it and thus burns fewer calories.

If you hike to your favorite waterfall as Kathleen does on Mondays, do some yoga on Tuesdays to sooth sore muscles and perhaps take a run or walk in the park with a friend on Wednesdays.

If you really love your Pilates class, do some basic Pilates for 15 minutes a day and then vary your routine with a brisk walk, some tai chi, free weight training or aerobics for the remainder of your exercise session.

I hike in the hills near my home several times a week and do yoga and weight training the other days.

We've both discovered that having a standing date for a walk or exercise class with a friend (or group of friends) every week is something we anticipate eagerly, plus it's an excellent source of inspiration and support. What a great way to visit—and you'll have no lunch calories to deal with!

So many of us women love to multitask and what better multitasking is there than combining your exercise session with a meditative state? We've discovered a series of tapes and CDs by Kelly Howell's BrainSync (www.brainsync.com) that does just that with a combination of great music, an energizing beat and sounds specifically designed to take you to a deeply meditative state so you can do exercise and soothe your mind at the same time.

How much exercise do you need? You've been faithfully doing your 20 minutes a day since Week 1, right? That's really the *minimum.*

The answer: Do as much as you can without overdoing. The more exercise you get, the healthier you will be. Harvard research shows that women who walk briskly at least half an hour three times a week reduce their risk of heart attacks by 40%. Increasing your brisk walking or aerobic time to four hours a week (that's only 35 minutes every day) provides a 50% reduction in heart attacks and a 50% protection against several types of cancer. Minimal exercise, at the rate of three 45-minute walks a week, proved to be enough to increase mental processing abilities by 20%, say University of Illinois researchers.

Ideally, go for 30 minutes a day four days a week of vigorous aerobic exercise, working hard enough to break into a light sweat. Schedule your workout for any time of day, as long as it's not within three hours of bedtime.

Then there is strength training. You can do it at a gym, with free weights at home, with Dynabands or even with Pilates and yoga. Muscle burns more calories than fat, so as you build muscle, you become more efficient at burning fat.

There are also dozens of ways you can get in a few minutes of exercise several times a day, and here are a few suggestions:

Jump. If you don't already have one, get a mini-trampoline. They're cheap, they're no impact, they don't take up much space, they're easy and fun to use, and they'll shake you up like nobody's business! In her book *The Fat Flush Plan* (McGraw-Hill, 2002), weight-loss expert Ann-Louise Gittleman recommends using a mini-trampoline to increase cardiovascular fitness, tone your body, fire up your cellular metabolism, energize your cells and best of all, get rid of toxins and cellulite by cleansing your lymphatic system.

Bike. Take a turn around the neighborhood before dinner. If that's not practical for you, buy an inexpensive exercise bike (thrift stores often sell them for less than $20) and ride every time you chat on the phone or watch the news on TV.

Watch TV. This means just the opposite of being a couch potato. Every time a commercial comes on (or even during a show, why not?), do a few lunges or ab crunches or squats. You'll get in at least 15 minutes of exercise an hour this way!

Go shopping. Of course, you know that parking farther away from the mall entrance will give you more walking time in the parking lot. Try walking all the way around the inside of the mall before you go into your first store. After you finish at one store, deliberately choose a store that's at the other end for your next stop. You may not be quite as efficient this way, but you'll get in lots of walking time. Use the stairs instead of the elevator.

Have moving meetings. If your business schedule is hectic, think about having walking meetings outside. You'll get a great deal done and get some exercise at the same time. Use the stairs at work instead of the elevator.

Change your social life. Does your social life involve spending a lot of time sitting in coffee shops or restaurants or movies with friends? Arrange to meet 20 minutes before your coffee date and take a brisk walk around the neighborhood before you sit down to sip java. Join an aerobics class with friends instead of going out for high-calorie meals. Instead of talking on the phone for hours, get together for a bike ride a couple of times a week. I have regular hiking dates with friends. We meet early in the morning before work and have a hike in the gorgeous nearby Santa Monica Mountains, complete with ocean views. It's a time to catch up, work out (there are some steep inclines), enjoy nature and even get some sunshine (not to be overdone, of course, but we need a certain amount to both produce vitamin D in our skin, and to stimulate our brains and hormonal systems).

Kathleen equally enjoys horseback riding with a friend or two in the forest a few minutes from her mountain home in North Carolina. Horseback riding has its particular challenges and sitting a horse correctly engages all the same core muscles as a Pilates workout.

Get creative! With this little boost, you'll be able to come up with your own ways to add a little exercise to your day. Think minute by minute. Flex your butt muscles while you brush your teeth (two minutes). Do arm circles while you talk on the phone. Do hip circles while you stir the soup. Your family might think you're off your rocker, but you'll be toning up beautifully! You'll find it's easy to get in an hour of exercise a day with all these mini-exercise sessions.

- Tense and release your thigh muscles when you're at a stoplight. Even better, do Kegel exercises. These repetitive contractions of your pelvic muscles keep that area in shape. Contract the muscles around your anus and vagina for a count of five, then release. Repeat five more times. Then repeat with shorter contractions to a count of one, and relax. Then repeat these short contractions five more times. This will prevent your uterus from dropping down with age (sorry, it does happen due to hormones and gravity), prevent urinary incontinence and is guaranteed to improve your sex life.

Here are some of our favorite exercise systems:

Pilates

We're big fans of this method of conditioning your body without punishing it. The Pilates method involves a series of exercises that place emphasis on building "core" strength through abdominal muscles and particularly the deepest muscles in your abdomen. This will help improve your balance and coordination and make other types of exercise easier.

In addition to building core strength, Pilates will help you get the strong, long, lean body of a dancer. Pilates combines movement with mental concentration and breath work, helping you feel physically, mentally and emotionally balanced. It's important to start with a qualified teacher, and we recommend a class taught by a certified Pilates instructor. Many teachers will invite you to sit in on a demonstration class. There are some excellent Pilates videos on the market such as those produced by Denise Austin and Elizabeth Larkam.

Yoga

We love yoga just as much as we enjoy Pilates, and Kathleen is a particular fan. She was a Kripalu yoga teacher for more than 30 years. Yoga is an ancient discipline that most often in Western practice involves stretching, flexibility, strength-building movements called "asanas," breathing exercises called "pranayama" and various forms of meditation and relaxation.

There are dozens of forms of yoga taught widely in the United States today, and each has its place. If you like a physical challenge and really want to feel the stretch and burn, you'd probably love power yoga, Iyengar, Bikram (hot) yoga or any of the vigorous varieties. If you'd prefer a gentle, rhythmic, meditative workout, you'll probably be happier with Kripalu yoga, white lotus yoga, gentle yoga, Vinyasa or flow yoga or any of the other gentle variations.

When you begin to practice yoga, be sure to move slowly and gently into the poses, stretching but not straining. Regardless of which method you choose (you might want to try two or three before actually signing up for a class), be sure you have a well-qualified teacher. As with Pilates, there are many yoga teachers with varying degrees of qualifications. Don't be afraid to ask questions.

There are also excellent yoga videos on the market today. We like these videos: Tracey Rich and Ganga White's Total Yoga series; Double Yoga by Ganga White; Kripalu Yoga—Gentle, Dynamic, and Partner series; and Lilias or Rodney Yee's numerous tapes. Yoga for Round Bodies is an excellent beginning tape for larger women.

DEALING WITH STRESS

We'll go much more deeply into the stress/lifestyle imbalance in Chapter 9, but because it is such a pervasive force in almost everyone's life, we want to give you some basics of stress management.

Most of us connect stress with the "not enough time" syndrome. We hurry to avoid being late to work, we hurry to meet deadlines, we hurry to meet friends so we can "relax and have fun," and most absurdly, we hurry to bed so we can get sufficient rest to do it all over again the next day.

We both confess we don't always take the time to de-stress, which leads to distress! When we do take the time, it makes a huge difference in our mental attitudes, physical strength, and productivity.

Do you have a lot of stress?

Imagine that you have an entire day alone, to do whatever you like. Here are the rules: No one else can be involved, and you can't do anything for anyone else. This is all about *you*.

What would you do?

Would you stay in your jammies all day and lounge on the couch drinking tea and reading a favorite book?

Would you walk through snowy woods or dig your toes into the sand of a peaceful beach?

Would you go for a long, solitary drive through the countryside?

Would you go to your favorite museum or browse in the library?

Would you paint a picture of the red maple in your backyard or write a poem about the first buds of spring?

If you're having difficulty imagining what you'd do on a day all to yourself, you're stressed. You'll benefit from the suggestions in this brief section and the more detailed discussion of stress management in Chapter 9.

For now, see if you can find a day to do exactly what you want to do this week. If a whole day isn't practical, see if you can set aside at least a couple of hours just for you.

Here are some other ways to get the stress monster under control.

Time Management

You might be surprised how quickly you can bring an end to time pressure and the stress that goes with it by keeping a "to-do" list. A simple pocket diary, a small desktop diary or even an electronic version will do the trick. First thing every morning, review what you *must* do that day. This includes appointments, deadlines, and so on. Make a list of them on a separate piece of paper that you can slip inside your schedule book or use the calendar function in your computer. Next, look at the things you would like to accomplish in the next few days. Choose one or two of those "want-to-do" things and add them to the "must-do" list. Finally, add one or two items from a "wish list" you've been keeping in a separate part of your schedule book.

It helps if you estimate how long each item will take so you don't overextend yourself. Give yourself the satisfaction of checking off each item as you accomplish it.

By organizing your schedule, you'll accomplish more, you'll do the things that are the most urgent, and you'll immediately know whether you can say yes to additional requests for your time. Most of all, you'll abolish the stress of trying to hold all of these things in your head.

Breathing

We talked about deep breathing in Chapter 1. If that's something that's slipped away from your daily practice, consider going back to it now. Your breathing and your emotions are intertwined. When your breathing is slow and deep, your emotions will be calm and cool and your stress will evaporate.

Exercise

Exercise is an excellent way of relieving stress, so you're already well on your way with your exercise program. If you're practicing yoga, you have made an especially good choice for stress relief.

Meditation

There are many excellent forms of meditation. Periods of quiet mind emptying are practiced by virtually every major religion as a means of contacting the creative forces of the universe. Meditation is a great stress reliever. Research from the Massachusetts Medical Center shows that meditators have lower levels of the stress hormone cortisol, plus meditation lowers your blood pressure, lowers your cholesterol, boosts your immune system and a host of other benefits.

Probably the simplest form of meditation is this:

- Close your eyes. Sit quietly and allow your breath to flow in and out.

- Focus all your attention on the breath.

- When thoughts come or your mind wanders, simply become aware of the shift and gently bring your focus back to your breath.

- Continue for 10 minutes or more.

Practicing this form of meditation (or any other form you like) first thing in the morning will bring you focus, balance, and calm. Any time you feel stressed, take five minutes to sit quietly in meditation to calm yourself.

Kathleen says when she worked in a hectic environment for a television network, she would go into the toilet stall, lock the door and just sit quietly for a few minutes to regain that feeling of calm.

Bonus tip: If you're feeling stressed, scattered, or unfocused during your day, try this simple grounding exercise:

Sitting in a chair or standing comfortably, imagine you have roots growing through the bottoms of your feet deep into the earth. Stretch your arms over your head and imagine you can reach all the way to the sky. Take three deep, slow breaths and visualize your body as perfectly balanced between earth and sky.

Aromatherapy

Smell affects us deeply and emotionally. Think of the smell of baking bread, the pine scents many of us associate with Christmas, the delicate scent of a rose or the salt tang of sea air.

Smells are carried directly to the part of the brain called the limbic system, a primitive part that acts as a kind of emotional switchboard that evaluates smells and directs corresponding emotional and physiological responses.

We remember smell longer than any other sensual input, so a particular scent can unlock and help us retrieve memories and in that way become a direct pathway to memory and emotion.

Fragrances can reduce stress and depression, relax or invigorate you, stimulate your sensory awareness and provide pain relief.

For aromatherapy or massage oils, it's important to buy good-quality natural essential oils labeled "100% pure" for maximum therapeutic value. You'll need to blend essential oils into carrier oils: refined, cold-pressed vegetable oils such as almond oil.

Here are a few favorites:

- For physical and emotional relaxation: lavender, chamomile, sandalwood, marjoram

- For mental clarity: eucalyptus, lemon

- For mood elevation: rose, geranium, bergamot

- For energy: eucalyptus, cinnamon, peppermint, clove, patchouli

You can use these oils individually or make your own blends to use in a bath, for a massage, for scenting a room, or even to apply as a perfume.

For more information on aromatherapy, go to www.aromaweb.com.

Massage

There's nothing quite like the pampered feeling your body, mind, and spirit get when you have a massage. A good massage therapist can drain the stress right out of you and leave you feeling relaxed yet alert and energized.

If a professional massage is out of your price range, ask your spouse or a friend to trade massages with you or buy one of the inexpensive massagers that are on the market now. It's even better if you use some of the aromatherapy oils mentioned in this chapter.

Acupressure

The ancient Chinese practice of acupressure can relieve stress and pain in a couple of minutes. It's a simple technique that involves applying fairly strong pressure to specific body points with your fingers.

TENSION-RELIEVING ACUPRESSURE POINTS

Neck: Place your hands behind your head, thumbs pointing downward, cradling the back of your head in the basket of your hands. Feel the thick cords of muscle that run up each side of your spine just under your skull. Use your thumbs to apply firm pressure to the two spots. Gently drop your head back into the pressure. When you feel a pulse on both sides, slowly release the pressure. This usually takes about a minute.

Shoulders: To release tension in your shoulders, press a point located in the highest point of your shoulder muscle. You'll find one or more very tender spots along the top of your shoulder, the trapezius muscle, and that's the right place. Sit in a comfortable chair and allow your body to relax. Let your head drop forward, breathe deeply, and, curving your fingers, apply firm pressure to the point for one minute. (Caution: Pregnant women should not use this point.)

Creative Therapy

Drawing, scribbling, doodling, writing a poem or dancing to African drumbeats all link you to the right side of your brain, the creative aspect of your being. Working on the right side of your brain eases stress and allows you to become more flexible in your viewpoint of whatever triggered the stress.

Journaling

You may have already found that you love your Wellness Journal. Many people tell us they continue their journals even after they've finished their Vibrant Health Plan. Journaling is a great way to unwind at the end of the day or to focus at the beginning of the day. You don't have to write the great American novel. It doesn't have to be in proper English and you don't have to stress about your spelling. Just let your feelings flow onto the paper. Some days you may feel like writing pages and pages. Other days a sentence or two will be all you need. Think of your journal as a place to confide your innermost thoughts, feelings and questions. Research shows that we can release emotions and resolve issues much better simply by writing them down in a journal and it can even enhance our immune systems and overall health.

FOR A MORE BEAUTIFUL YOU

If skin, hair, and beauty issues are a concern for you, what you're already doing will go a long way toward restoring glowing, toned skin, silky hair and a sparkle in your eyes. Exercise, a better diet, more water, and stress management are your best friends. But there are some more specific things you can do to feel and look better.

Skin

Of course you know that wearing sunscreen is essential for preventing sun damage, so you're wearing a moisturizer or makeup that includes sunscreen every time you go out of the house, right? Right.

A great moisturizer—one that is the right moisturizer for your skin—will go a long way toward preventing wrinkles and plumping up your skin to erase those fine lines. We love creams that include bovine colostrum, alpha lipoic acid, and/or ester-C and coenzyme Q_{10} among other skin-healing supplements.

I live in a very dry part of the country and need a good cream to stave off the wrinkles. My favorite night cream contains the antioxidants vitamin C, alpha lipoic acid, vitamin E and coenzyme Q_{10}. It's rejuvenating, stays moist in a dewy way and makes my skin feel and look great. It also does not contain any harmful chemical additives. Many people don' t realize that these additives are absorbed through the skin.

Wrinkling, acne and dry skin are caused by inflammation, which causes all kinds of problems throughout your system ranging from the breakdown of collagen that makes skin plump and smooth to arthritis and even heart disease. Limiting your intake of inflammation-causing foods such as red meat, refined sugars, and processed foods will contribute to lovely skin as well as vibrant health.

Beyond these basic beauty tips, adding essential fatty acids and antioxidants to your diet will be great for your skin. Essential fatty acids are healthy oils like flaxseed, fish, soy, canola, and olive oils.

Antioxidants are the "good guys" that neutralize a process called oxidation in your system. Think of a sliced apple: when you leave it on the counter for a few minutes, it will begin to turn brown because of oxidation.

When this takes place in your body, as it does every day because of exposure to pollutants in your environment, poor nutritional choices and the natural aging process, cells don't reproduce perfectly and you get wrinkles, heart disease and even cancer. Antioxidants, which are present in all fruits and vegetables and in dozens of great supplements, stop that oxidation process and keep you healthy.

In addition to the 64 ounces of water you're drinking, be sure you eat at least three modest-sized meals a day and two snacks, one at mid-morning and the other at mid-afternoon, eating protein first. Each snack must contain protein, carbohydrate and fat in the form of essential omega-3 and omega-6 fatty acids. For example: a slice of turkey, half a dozen nuts and half an apple *or* two ounces of feta cheese mixed with half a dozen Greek olives packed in olive oil and half a pear *or* two ounces of tuna, two small whole grain crackers and four grape tomatoes.

This simple dietary change will help plump up your skin and improve your resistance to skin-damaging environmental pollutants. They'll also help control the cravings that lead to unhealthy eating and weight gain.

Hair

All of the previous recommendations will improve hair texture and moisture as well. Probably the most effective will be the addition of healthy fats into your diet.

As we age, hair often thins in response to waning estrogen levels, so consider reading Chapters 11 and 12 on hormone and thyroid imbalances and perhaps adding some natural phytoestrogens to your supplement arsenal, even if thinning hair isn't your major concern.

FINALLY

Break out of your routine; try something you've never done before. Get a massage or a facial. Discover a beautiful natural area nearby that you haven't explored before. Share the fun with a friend. You may find something that becomes a passion for you.

This is your time to explore and have fun while you do it!

8

WEEK 8

Where You Are
and Where You're Going

EVALUATE YOUR PROGRESS

Congratulations! You're in the final week of your Vibrant Health Plan. We hope you know much more about yourself and your health than you did just eight short weeks ago and that you have the tools at your fingertips to find any other information you need.

Undoubtedly your Wellness Journal is filled with useful information: Websites you've found in your own research, links and articles you've run across that helped you so far on this journey. This information will come in handy again, whether you're reassessing your own health or helping a friend find her way back to health.

Now is the time to evaluate your progress. Even if you were already practicing a healthy lifestyle, we hope we've been able to offer you new ideas. And we hope that you've made substantial progress toward understanding and addressing the underlying imbalances that were causing your symptoms.

You've no doubt discovered that unraveling the mysteries of the human body and the imbalances that cause health problems is a painstaking and complex process. There may be blind alleys and false starts. There is no one-size-fits-all prescription for systemic imbalances, and many problems take time to treat.

This week we'll give you some tools to help you determine if you've chosen the right path and if you're heading in the right direction—toward health.

DO THE QUESTIONNAIRE AGAIN

Fill in your current answers to items on the original questionnaire.

Now compare your answers to when you first did the questionnaire during Week 2.

What's different? Take a red pen and mark the answers that are different in the two versions. A pattern should begin to emerge.

Perhaps you've discovered that your major symptoms have changed and that your imbalances are beginning to be corrected. Perhaps some have disappeared. Perhaps some imbalances have shifted to other areas.

Think of these two versions of your questionnaire as a road map. Look backward and you can see where you've been; look forward and you'll begin to get an idea of where you need to go.

WHAT'S WORKED FOR YOU

List the major symptoms you listed in Week 2: _____

On a scale of 1 to 10, 10 being the best, rate the severity of these symptoms today: _____

Have any of your symptoms become more severe?   ❏ Yes   ❏ No

If no, just keep on doing what you're doing now. It's working!
If yes, continue from here:

Which symptoms have worsened? _____

_____

Have some parts of the Vibrant Health Plan been difficult for you?   ❏ Yes   ❏ No

If yes, which ones? _____

_____

Why were they difficult? _____

_____

What can you do to effectively replace the difficult task? (If cravings are still a problem, take another look at Chapter 6.) _____

_____

_____

Are you willing to try something different to address your difficulty?
Yes _____ No _____

Take a break now and reread Chapter 4. Work through the "Decision Tree" again.

Is there another imbalance that jumps out at you?   Yes _____ No _____

If yes, which one? _____

What makes you think this imbalance could be causing the symptoms you are experiencing right now? _____

_____

What is your personal plan to address this? _____

_____

_____

Now re-read the chapter on the new imbalance you are considering.

Does this trigger some recognition in you?   Yes _____ No _____

If your answer is "yes," start working the Vibrant Health Plan again with this new imbalance.

If your answer is "no," try this:

Spend at least 15 minutes doing your breathing exercises and meditation. Now start over with rereading Chapter 4 and working the "Decision Tree" again. Getting into a meditative state will actually help you clear your mind, focus better, and tap into your natural intuition.

You might also try tuning in to your inner voice (see Chapter 4) and ask questions that will lead you toward better balance.

You will eventually hit on the exact mix for you. It takes perseverance, courage, intuition, and a positive attitude, but you'll find it! Have faith in yourself, and vibrant health will be your reward.

FEELING STUCK?

You may be progressing more slowly than you would like. We'd all prefer instant gratification! We have grown up in a world of quick fixes. Some of the brain chemistry imbalances we have mentioned can be corrected in days. Blood sugar and hormonal imbalances can often be corrected fairly quickly. But other imbalances may take time to correct, so please be patient.

Many supplements take time to act because they're working throughout your system to restore balance rather than simply addressing symptoms. If you've suffered from headaches, an aspirin or a Tylenol may make the pain go away temporarily. But the pain will keep on returning until you address the cause of your headaches. You've done a lot of work to discover the cause of your health problem, so take the time to refine and restructure your plan.

Each chapter in Part 2 offers numerous ways of addressing particular imbalances. We certainly don't expect you'll do them all and likely you've done some picking and choosing along the way.

If you extend this program for another few weeks and you still feel stuck, try something different. Try some of the other suggestions in your imbalances section. For example, if you were working through the sex hormone imbalances section and you used black cohosh and other herbs for perimenopausal symptoms without the results you were hoping for, you might want to consider prescription natural hormone replacement. You'll need to enlist your doctor's support for this.

You might want to look at a different area of imbalance altogether and work through the Vibrant Health Plan again, this time focusing on it. For example, Nina thought her allergies and chemical sensitivities might be related to dysbiosis and candida overgrowth, but after working through this plan and the information in Chapter 14, she still had some symptoms. One problem was fatigue that became worse when she was around certain odorous chemicals, such as new fabrics or gasoline. She took a closer look at Chapter 15 and decided to do a hair analysis. It came back with high mercury levels and was confirmed by a urine "heavy metal provocation test." Mercury can create havoc in many parts of the body, including fostering hard- to treat yeast (candida) infections.

If you choose to go to another imbalance chapter, work through the weekly assignments again just as you did the first time. Consider different testing to cast more light on your condition.

It's important that you persevere. Eventually, you'll find the combination that works for you. Remember, there is not one solution that works for every individual. You and your body are unique, so your detective work with the Vibrant Health Plan is a key to finding your own personal solution. Eventually, you'll have success.

It's your choice. It's your health. And you can do it!

Now is the time to integrate what's worked best for you and to translate this short-term plan into a longer-term approach for a long and healthy life.

YOUR LONG-TERM VIBRANT HEALTH PLAN

Even though this is the last week of your Vibrant Health Plan, it's not in any way the end of your quest for better health. In fact, you've just begun.

We hope these eight weeks of exploring your health have helped you take the first steps toward a new life and a new lifestyle. We also hope you have addressed the major symptoms that led you to seek better balance in the first place and that you've had success in uncovering the underlying imbalances that caused the symptoms.

If you've carefully followed the Vibrant Health Plan, we know you're feeling more energized and less stressed. We'd love to hear about your experiences. Please write us at www.drcass.com and at www.kathleenbarnes.com. We've been honored to share this journey with you!

2

ADDRESSING
THE IMBALANCES
THAT ARE
MAKING YOU SICK

9

DE-STRESS
YOUR LIFE

I t is almost impossible to exist in today's world without stress. We all feel it: The pressures of job, home, kids, health, finances. It goes on and on. And now we're lucky enough to have cell phones, so your office, your kids, your spouse, your best friend in crisis, your child's teacher . . . You name it, stress can reach you any time, any place.

Every day, our personal time shrinks. We consider it an indulgence if we can squeeze in the time to simply sit and enjoy a cup of tea, read a book for the sheer pleasure of it or take a long, leisurely bubble bath. Never before in history have humans had so much to do and so many varieties of ways to do it. Even sitting around the television set at night with your family can be stress producing with so many channels from which to choose (and deciding who gets to choose them!) and then watching shows with so much fast-paced and violent action.

We rarely get a chance to catch our breath. And it's taking a huge toll on our health.

The American Psychological Association estimates that 75% of all visits to primary care physicians are for stress-related problems, and surveys show 75% of us have reported we feel "great stress" at least one day a week. A 2007 study by the American Psychological Association shows that more than one-third of Americans suffer extreme stress on a daily basis.

Even our kids feel the pressure to participate in half a dozen after-school activities, and, as young as the age of nine, they're already feeling pressure to work harder and do more in order to get into the "right" college.

Unfortunately, unresolved stress in your life can lead to a downward spiral of depression and anxiety and cause a wide range of physical problems from headaches and heart disease to weight gain, gastrointestinal problems, and more.

If this is all ringing true with you, you're not alone. Here's a story that may seem familiar.

Ashley, a 35-year-old real estate agent, single parent, and self-styled "soccer mom," was the first to acknowledge her life was filled with stress. "I know I'm stressed, and I know my headaches are related, but I just don't know how to break this vicious cycle," she told me. I could see she was already paying the price of her stress with weight gain, frequent colds and chronic tiredness.

THE CAUSES OF STRESS

First of all, as I told Ashley, stress isn't always bad. It can be a motivator. It's what gets you out of bed in the morning and sends you to the office or for your semiannual dental checkup. But when stress takes over your life and when you're unable to release it, it sets up a toxic cycle that can make you sick.

You may have taken some of those stress-indicator questionnaires that run from time to time in women's magazines or get sent around on the Internet. They vary in their methods and questions, but it's true that the emotional stress of generally happy life events such as having a baby, getting married, buying a new house or getting a promotion can have the same physiological effects as dealing with the major illness of a close member of your family, losing a job or having a family member in jail.

The stress itself is not the issue. Stress is in our lives whether we like it or not. The real question is this: How do you deal with stress? We have included the well-researched Homes-Rahe scale here, to help you evaluate the recent stressful events in your life and the toll they might take on your health.

THE COST OF STRESS

Until you find a way to resolve and release your stress, you're creating a vicious cycle that can cause serious damage to your health in the long run.

LIFE STRESS QUESTIONNAIRE

Have you had any of the following things happen to you during the past year? Jot down the numbers following each of the events you've experienced, and add them up to get your grand total.

LIFE EVENT	POINT VALUE
Change in social activities	15
Change in sleeping habits	15
Change in residence	20
Change in work hours	20
Change in church activities	20
Tension at work	25
Small children in the home	25
Change in living conditions	25
Outstanding personal achievement	30
Problem teenager(s) in the home	30
Trouble with in-laws	30
Difficulties with peer group	30
Son or daughter leaving home	30
Change in responsibilities at work	30
Taking over major financial responsibility	30
Foreclosure of mortgage or loan	30
Change in relationship with spouse	35
Change to different line of work	35
Loss of a close friend	35
Gain of a new family member	40
Sexual difficulties	40
Pregnancy	40
Change in health of family member	45
Retirement	45

Loss of job	50
Change in quality of religious faith	50
Marriage	50
Personal injury or illness	50
Loss of self-confidence	60
Death of a close family member	60
Injury to reputation	60
Trouble with the law	65
Marital separation	65
Divorce	75
Death of a spouse	100
Grand total	____

Your total score measures the amount of stress to which you have been subjected. A score of 150 or less is just about the normal level most of us deal with on an ongoing basis. Continue reading this chapter for some suggestions on handling your stress even better. With a score of 150 to 250, you're seriously stressed and most likely are experiencing the effects of toxic stress. You'll certainly benefit from the Vibrant Health Plan in this chapter. If you scored 250 to 300, you're clearly in a stress-overload situation, and the information in this chapter will help you regain your ability to cope. Above a score of 350, you are seriously stressed and need to take action with all the resources this chapter offers—now. If your score is over 350, you might consider seeking professional help through this difficult time in your life.

Unresolved stress, the kind of stress you haven't dealt with and eliminated from your body and mind, is sometimes called *chronic* or *toxic stress*. This sustained stress overrides your body's natural abilities to bounce back. Stress keeps piling upon stress, leaves stress hormones at high levels and suppresses your immune system, leaving you vulnerable to colds, flu, and all kinds of illnesses.

We don't want to scare you, but this fact has been scientifically validated: People who are diagnosed with various types of cancer have frequently undergone a recent major life stress, such as the breakup of a marriage, a bankruptcy or the illness or death of a close family member.

Our responses to stress are ancient and instinctive. When we think we are in danger in some way, our adrenal glands release adrenaline. This increases breathing and heart rates and sends extra blood sugar to the muscles in preparation to fight or flee from the threat of physical danger. This "fight-or-flight" response worked just fine when our ancestors were fleeing from saber-toothed tigers.

However, that protection mechanism doesn't serve us very well today when the threats are far more often mental and emotional. After all, you can't run away from your desk, your ringing telephone, your sick child or your boss' insistence that you work overtime. You may grumble, growl or grit your teeth, but the stress response remains unreleased and the next phase sets in. Your adrenals now release cortisol, the hormone of chronic stress, in an attempt to shore you up. For more information on the adrenal glands, see Chapter 12.

In his book *Waking the Tiger* (North Atlantic Books, 1997), psychologist Peter Levine describes the coping mechanisms of wild animals. When they've been stressed, animals instinctively go through a series of movements to disperse the energy and complete the stress cycle. Modern-day humans seem to have forgotten how to do this. Thus, this toxic stress stays inside us, exacting a high price.

Toxic stress diminishes your body's ability to produce cortisol and another adrenal hormone, DHEA (dehydroepiandrosterone), when you need them. You become even less able to respond in an appropriate way to stressors and to end the stress cycle.

Here are some of the prices you pay for toxic stress in the short term:

- Suppressed immune system, increasing risk of infections
- Reduced rate of body's ability to repair itself
- Slower metabolism
- Reduced ability to absorb vital nutrients

You may experience the following symptoms:

- Recurring headaches
- Vague aches and pains
- Dizziness
- Heartburn

- Muscle tension

- Dry mouth

- Excessive perspiration

- Pounding heart

- Insomnia

- Fatigue

The long-term price you pay is even heavier:

- Acceleration of the aging process

- Weight gain

- Increased risk of digestive problems (ulcers, colitis), osteoporosis, high blood pressure, heart disease, and even cancer

Emotionally, when your brain runs out of the feel-good brain chemicals, you experience the following:

- Anxiety, fear, restlessness

- Irritability, anger

- Depression

- Insecurity

- Loss of sex drive

- Excessive eating, smoking, drinking, or drug use

There's another important mechanism that takes place when you are chronically stressed: your blood sugar levels rise and then abruptly fall. That's because adrenaline and cortisol dump sugar into your bloodstream, and in an hour or two your blood sugar crashes. This is a serious problem because 20% of your body's entire intake of glucose fuels your brain, so when your sugars crash, you start feeling foggy, nervous, tired, and irritable. Your instinct, like Ashley's, is to reach for a doughnut, Coke, or cup of coffee, so you feel "up" for an hour or so before the cycle begins again. Ashley began to recognize that the toxic downward spiral was causing her headaches, colds and flu and even weight gain.

WE'RE ALL ADRENALINE JUNKIES

Have you ever heard of adrenaline junkies—the kind of folks who love extreme sports, who are always looking for the next "rush"? The sad truth is, almost all of us are adrenaline junkies in one way or another.

Even if you're not a bungee jumper or extreme skier, you might recognize yourself in Ashley's experience. She decided to take a week off and go to the beach, hang out, read books, eat seafood and just relax. What happened?

"After two days, I was jumping out of my skin," she told me. "I couldn't sit still, I couldn't focus on the novel I was reading and I just wanted to get up and *do* something."

Does this sound familiar? Ashley was experiencing adrenaline withdrawal. She had become so addicted to the constant flow of adrenaline, she didn't know what to do when it stopped. She was willing to do anything, even go back to the city and the sources of all her stressors, to get it to start up again.

Beyond our present day stresses, we actually store mental images of traumatic events for many years. They can pop up again in response to a trigger of a similar situation or just out of the blue. When they do, our bodies respond exactly as they did to the initial stressor.

To make matters worse, we 21st-century humans stress and worry about things that haven't happened yet or things that might happen someday or might never happen at all. How many times have you stayed awake at night worrying about paying a bill? How many times have you fretted and stewed over a job interview or your child's recital or a presentation at work?

As Mark Twain once said, "I have lived a long life and had many troubles . . . most of which never happened."

RECOGNIZING STRESS IN YOUR LIFE

There are dozens of ways to get your stress monster under control. The key to managing stress is recognizing when you're experiencing it, taking action to break the stress cycle, and using long-term methods to keep it from spiraling out of control.

How can you recognize stress? It's become such a pervasive part of our lives that most of us think this is a normal way of living. Here are some signs of immediate stress that you can recognize:

- Muscle tension

- Irregular breathing

- Pounding heart

- Butterflies in stomach

- Agitation

- Irritability

- Sudden flush

Tests

See Chapter 12 for information on testing the adrenal glands.

DEALING WITH STRESS

We all need to learn how to stop the stress cycle and rest, recover, and rebuild ourselves—every day, if necessary.

The solution for many has been to find relief by turning to drink, downers, or dope, all of which have their own destructive effects. These substances promote the release of the feel-good neurotransmitter dopamine plus endorphins, which make you feel high, and GABA (gamma-aminobutyric acid), the relaxing neurotransmitter. Yet booze, pills and pot can throw your neurotransmitter and blood sugar levels out of balance, causing all kinds of trouble ranging from emotional and mental imbalance to addiction and withdrawal.

Happily, there are natural choices that will help you break the cycle safely and without side effects.

Our lives cannot be completely free of stress, but we can control how we respond to it. by following these steps, we can break the toxic stress cycle and restore our natural ability to release stress: :

- Balance blood sugar

- Promote the release of GABA

- Support the release of dopamine and endorphins

- Supply the appropriate nutrients to produce them

Conventional Medical Treatment

Although at least 75% of visits to doctors' offices are due to stress-related illness, conventional medicine has nothing to offer besides symptomatic care. And that is only once you have actually developed a "real" illness, whether it's high blood pressure, ulcers, migraine headaches, back pain, or diabetes. The best way to handle stress-related illness is prevention.

Lifestyle

Take some time to reflect on your diet and lifestyle.

Are you getting enough sleep? Lack of quality sleep can make you cranky and irritable. It can even raise your blood pressure and cause physiological stress.

Is your diet optimal for good health? As we mentioned in earlier chapters, you should eliminate processed foods, especially refined sugar, from your diet. Consider withdrawing (gradually if necessary) from caffeine to eliminate a big-time dietary stressor. Eat high-quality protein from seafood, poultry, lean meats, soy, beans and whole grains to keep your blood sugar stable.

To change her lifestyle, Ashley first decided to begin saying "no" to requests for more volunteer work at her son's school and she asked that her business partner share the workload more evenly. They worked out a better schedule so that she had more time off. She then stopped eating on the run. She began to eat three meals a day, starting with a protein shake to which she added some fruit and a tablespoon of flax oil and a midmorning and afternoon snack of fruit, cheese, or veggies. Her overall energy immediately began to improve, without the daily dips.

She added high-quality omega-3 "good" fats from sources like salmon and tuna and omega-6 from vegetable oils. These essential fatty acids (EFAs) are especially important for stress and related disorders because they support the activity of neurotransmitters, particularly serotonin. Fats make up 60% of the brain's weight and these essential fats promote healthy brain cell communication, powerfully affecting your mind and mood.

Natural Stress Relief

Here are some herbs and supplements that are effective stress busters and energy rebuilders.

Kava (*piper methysticum*): Long in use in the South Pacific as a relaxing social beverage, kava has a role to play in today's stressful world.

Research shows the kava works as well as the benzodiazepines (Valium, Ativan, Halcion, Klonopin, Xanax etc) without the potential for addiction and the serious side effects associated with the prescription drugs. These include drowsiness, nausea, depression, sleep disturbances, memory loss and increased potential for having accidents.

Unlike prescription drugs that require ever-increasing doses to get the same effect, there are no withdrawal symptoms if you decide to quit taking kava. A low daytime dose will relax you without making you sleepy. In larger doses, kava will help you sleep without a morning hangover. In fact, kava has long been known to enhance concentration while helping you stay relaxed.

Kava acts on the limbic system, the emotional center of the brain, and directly on the muscles. In addition to relieving stress, the muscle-relaxing effect makes it helpful for headaches, backaches and other tension-related pain.

Kava's precise effect on neurotransmitters is not fully understood, but it appears to enhance the receptivity of the brain's calming GABA receptors.

You can get kava in tablets, capsules or tinctures. Read the label to determine the amount of kavalactones, the active ingredient, are in the product you are purchasing.

Cautions: Despite its excellent safety record, in 2002, kava came under question by the U.S. Food and Drug Administration based on European reports it may cause liver damage. However, a large number of published safety and toxicity studies clearly indicate that kava is far safer, and less liver toxic, than conventional anti-anxiety and antidepressant prescription drugs. In fact, the leading single cause of liver failure in Western countries is overdose of the common pain medication, acetaminophen (Tylenol).

In conclusion, we all need to be aware that all herbs are potent medicines and should be treated with appropriate respect.

If you decide to take kava, please follow these guidelines:

Don't use it if you have liver disease or if you are a heavy alcohol user.

Don't exceed a maximum of 250 mg of kavalactones per day.

Taken at these levels, kava has only mild side effects, including occasional skin rashes, headache or mild stomach upset.

Dosage: 60–75 mg of kavalactones, the usual capsule dosage size, taken two to three times daily.

With a 30% standardized extract, you'll need 200–300 mg per dose.

If you're using kava to aid sleep, take your daily dosage all at once, 45 minutes before bedtime.

Valerian: Sometimes referred to as "Nature's Valium," valerian is very effective for treating stress. It's a natural relaxant that combats nervousness, insomnia, restlessness and depression. Like kava, it acts on the GABA receptors to produce a calming effect similar to that of valium without the side effects.

Be forewarned : The smell of valerian has been likened to old socks or worse, so you'll probably prefer taking it in capsule or tablet form.

Cautions: Valerian increases the effects of other sedative drugs, including muscle relaxants and antihistamines. It can interact negatively with alcohol, narcotics and other psychotropic drugs.

Dosage: To promote relaxation, 50–100 mg two or three times a day. To help you sleep, take 150–400 mg 45 minutes before bedtime. Look for standardized product with 0.8% valeric acid.

Theanine: This amino acid has sometimes been called "Zen in a bottle" for its unique ability to chill you out in a hurry, giving you that sense of alert calmness. Theanine, (chemically referred to as L-theanine) is a major ingredient in green tea, taken for centuries by Asian monks to keep them calm but awake during their meditations. Theanine increases the relaxed, yet focused "alpha" state of the brain, measurable by an electroencephalograph (EEG). Theanine works by increasing your body's levels of the calming neurotransmitter GABA (gamma amino butyric acid).

Cautions: None at the recommended dosage.

Dosage: Take 100–200 mg twice daily. Can be taken with GABA for enhanced effect.

GABA (gamma-aminobutyric acid): Known as the "cool" neurotransmitter, GABA has a dampening effect on the central nervous system and controls the release of the stimulating dopamine in the reward center of the brain. Anxiety, tension and insomnia, are associated with low GABA levels, while adequate levels help you to feel tranquil. Valium is a GABA-enhancing drug, but you can take GABA in supplement form without the side effects (and high cost!) of the prescription drug.

Cautions: Can cause nausea at high doses.
Dosage: 100–500 mg one to three times daily between meals.

Magnesium: The mineral, magnesium is involved in more than 300 body processes, including helping your body assimilate calcium and vitamin D, essential for healthy bones and a variety of other critical body processes. Often deficient in diabetics, magnesium also improves insulin's ability to transport glucose into cells. Magnesium has a direct effect on serotonin balance and helps keep us calm and relaxed. It provides relief for both migraine and tension headaches.
Cautions: Excessive magnesium acts as a laxative and may cause diarrhea at high doses. Use chelated forms such as magnesium aspartate, glycinate or citrate, which are absorbed and utilized more efficiently than the more common (and less expensive) magnesium oxide. Magnesium has (rarely) been associated with drops in blood sugar.
Dosage: Take 200–400 mg up to three times daily. Take the last dose at bedtime. To increase absorption, be sure to get 30–50 mg of Vitamin B_6. For migraines, take 500–1,000 mg daily as prevention.

Glutamine (also called L-glutamine): As a precursor to GABA, this amino acid has a calming effect in the brain. It's absorbed quickly and will give you an almost instant pick-me-up similar to a longed-for stimulant, including food or alcohol. In fact, as mentioned on page 77, a capful under your tongue will stop cravings for sugar and alcohol, as well as other substances. The most common amino acid found in muscle tissues, glutamine improves mental energy and relaxation, reduces addiction, stabilizes blood sugar and promotes memory. Glutamine naturally elevates levels of growth hormone in your body, making your cells multiply faster and slowing aging. Additional amounts of growth hormone help mobilize fat from storage, and make it available for energy.
Cautions: Do not use if you have kidney or liver disease.
Dosage: Take up to four 500 mg capsules daily with your regular supplements or add glutamine powder to a protein drink (without added sugar). It's best taken about 30 minutes before a meal for fat management or at bedtime to enhance growth hormone production.

Taurine: A non-essential amino acid, taurine enhances the activity of GABA and reduces irritability, insomnia, migraines and depression. Taurine helps move potassium, sodium, calcium and magnesium in and out of cells, helping generate nerve impulses, stabilize nerve cell membranes and prevent erratic firing of nerve cells. Taurine is very concentrated in the brain and it has been used to control epilepsy and other excitable brain states, including stress and anxiety, since it functions as a mild sedative. I have also prescribed it for bipolar patients to help prevent manic episodes.

Cautions: May lower blood pressure.

Dosage: Take 250–500 mg twice daily, between meals.

B-vitamins: Stress, exhaustion and anxiety actually deplete your supply of B-vitamins, since they are used in making the stress hormones and neurotransmitters. B-vitamins play a critical role in helping energy levels on an even keel and replenishing energy when it is depleted. These essential vitamins work in close combination to influence a wide variety of body processes. They are vital for delivering oxygen to the brain and protecting it from harmful oxidants. They also help turn glucose into energy within brain cells and help to keep neurotransmitters in circulation. They also support correct nerve function and stop the over-reactive neuron firing that results from emotional stress. There are 17 B vitamins and you need them all, every day. While there is no one food that contains all 17, fish, nuts, dairy products, soy, enriched whole grains and pork are good sources of B vitamins.

Cautions: None at the recommended dosages. It's best to take a complete B-complex for the optimal balance. If you take extra B_6, make sure you also take equivalent doses of the other B vitamins to prevent (reversible) neurological problems.

Dosage: Look for B-complex than contains at least 20 mg of niacin (vitamin B_3), 20 mg of vitamin B_6, 100 mcg. of folic acid, 100 mcg. of vitamin B_{12} and 50 mg of pantothenic acid (vitamin B_5). For best absorption, you'll also need at least 50 mg of magnesium, which is often deficient in our diets and helps to keep you calm.

In addition to her regular supplement program, I suggested that Ashley take my CALM Natural Mind Formula, a combination of theanine, GABA, glutamine, taurine, hops, passionflower and lemon balm, with B vitamins and magnesium. Within a week, she felt calmer, more focused, and no longer jittery. She also reported that her headaches were infrequent and far milder, and she was sleeping better. She was actually looking forward to a trip to Disneyland with her son, when a few short weeks earlier she would have dreaded it.

MORE WAYS TO APPROACH STRESS

Yoga

We talked about yoga and its universal benefits in Chapter 7. We believe yoga is one of the best long-term ways of addressing the stresses of modern life.

If you're looking specifically for stress relief, choose hatha yoga, the practice of specific movements, breathing exercises and meditation. The slower, calmer varieties of yoga, like Kripalu yoga, emphasize deliberate and meditative movement. Don't be fooled by the slow, contemplative pace. You'll get a great workout, while your stressed-out mind will get a break, You will leave class feeling both energized and relaxed.

Exercise

We already talked about exercise in Chapter 7. We'd now like to reinforce the idea that exercise is a great safety valve. A good run on the beach or a game of tennis or a bun-burning aerobic workout with your favorite video or in a gym helps let off the excess pressure. It actually helps your body break the acute

---

30-SECOND STRESS BUSTER

Breathe! Whenever you feel any of the symptoms of stress, stop and take three full, deep, slow breaths. This is an instant short-term fix. It will give you time to think, to rebalance, and to slow down and respond rather than unthinkingly react to the stressor.

You can find the best technique for deep breathing in Chapter 1.

It's important that your breathing is slow and relaxed. In just a minute or two, you'll feel your racing mind beginning to slow down, your mental clarity returning and the physical symptoms beginning to fade. Your brain has been oxygenated, producing a natural oxygen high and, most importantly, you've taken a big step toward breaking the toxic stress cycle.

stress cycle and allows your body and your hormonal system to reset and return to balance.

Stress responds to exercise better than does nearly any other condition. Exercise actually reduces the amount of adrenal hormones your body releases in response to stress and helps raise the level of mood-elevating endorphins in your brain.

Meditation

You cannot control the world around you, but regular meditation can help you control your reactions to it. Meditation isn't some esoteric Eastern practice; it's actually an integral part of virtually every world religion. It differs from prayer, however, in the sense that meditation is not "asking," it's "listening." It helps you find a way above the turbulence of daily life and it just might help awaken you to the "big picture" in which everything in life falls into place.

By slowing your mind's chatter, you automatically become calmer and more focused. Meditation has scientifically researched benefits to your body, not the least of which is better responsiveness to stressful events and quicker recovery from the physiological aspects of stress. In fact, researchers at the University of Massachusetts Medical Center found that meditators have lower levels of the stress hormone cortisol.

Considering what we now know about the "fight-or-flight" response and our out-of-whack stress reactions, meditation can help bring you back into balance and keep you from reacting to every tiny little stressor as though that saber-toothed tiger was hot on your tail.

Most meditation techniques involve physical relaxation combined with focusing on one thing, such as your breath, a lighted candle, or a mantra, such as "Om," or "One."

In time, and with practice, most meditators find themselves experiencing an expanded state of awareness in which the mind becomes still, the body relaxes, and emotions settle. This is not an imagined state. It's induced by changes in brain waves that take you from high-activity beta waves to a slower, calmer, focused alpha rhythm and eventually to a theta state, almost a trancelike state of deep relaxation from which arise many creative thoughts and ideas.

We're including one simple meditation technique here for you to try.

BASIC MEDITATION

Find a quiet place. Turn off your phone. Wear loose, comfortable clothing, or loosen your clothing so you are completely comfortable. You may want a shawl or blanket over your shoulders because body temperatures tend to drop as you relax.

Find a comfortable seated posture with your spine straight. It's fine to sit in a chair, but if you do, be sure your feet are flat on the floor. If you're sitting on the floor, tuck a firm cushion under your pelvis to help you keep your spine comfortably straight.

Consciously relax tension in your body. Pay particular attention to relaxing your shoulders, belly, and jaw.

Begin to take deep, slow breaths through your nose, relaxing your belly as you inhale and gently contracting the abdominal muscles as you exhale. Do this for at least nine breaths.

Now let your breath find its own rhythm. Keep your awareness on the simple inhalation and exhalation.

If your mind wanders, bring it back to the breath without mental comment. If you realize you've been distracted for some time, repeat the nine deep belly breaths and begin again.

Continue this for at least 10 minutes every day. If you like, you can set a timer on your watch so you don't have to distract yourself with time concerns. Meditation early in the morning gives you a good and focused start to your day, but you can certainly repeat it any time you feel the need.

Acupressure

As we mentioned in Chapter 7, acupressure is a wonderful do-it-yourself part of traditional Chinese medicine. It works on energy meridians in the body in much the same way acupuncture works, but without the needles! By simply pressing key points on the surface of your skin, you'll be stimulating your body's natural self-healing abilities. Applying firm but gentle pressure to specific points, you can release muscle tension and promote the circulation of blood and the body's life force energy to aid healing. The healing touch of acupressure reduces tension, increases circulation, and enables deep physical relaxation. Best of all, you can stimulate most acupressure points yourself by applying pressure with your fingers, knuckles, a pencil eraser, or similar item for a length of time ranging from 20 seconds to a couple of minutes.

Acupressure points can be very generalized, like the one called "Shen men," located at the crease of your wrist on the side opposite the thumb. Find the tender point and gently apply pressure for about a minute. Repeat on the other hand. It is known in traditional Chinese medicine to calm the spirit and regulate and tone the heart.

If acupressure piques your interest, re-read the acupressure section of Chapter 7.

Others

There are many other stress-relieving modalities, including massage, chi gong, tai chi, drumming, singing and chanting, to name just a few. Explore them, and find what works for you.

Two months after she started to address her toxic stress Ashley's yoga class had become her passion. Not only had she effortlessly lost the 10 excess pounds that were plaguing her, she had been headache free for a month and was sleeping peacefully through the night.

You may protest that you don't have time to do these exercises or techniques. However, you don't have time *not* to do them! You will be far more productive and far happier when you include them in your daily schedule.

10

BALANCING YOUR
BRAIN CHEMISTRY

B rain chemistry is the link between mind and body. In this chapter, you'll
get some tools to help you better understand your brain chemistry, the
mind-body connection and the relationship between mental health and physical well-being.

Depression, anxiety, panic, obsessions, addictions and memory loss are too
often considered to be a matter of "mind over matter." Friends, family, and
sadly, even therapists will tell you that self-discipline or extensive psychotherapy are the ways to kick these mind-states. Or they may urge you to take a prescription medication.

The news is this: Rather that being crazy, neurotic or hopelessly psychologi-
cally damaged, you may simply be deficient in certain nutrients!
Most mainstream medical practitioners overlook the fact that mood, behavior,
and mental performance all depend on your balance of neurotransmitters, the
chemical messengers of the brain. It's not simply mind over matter, but can also
be matter over mind!

The keys to your brain function are the chemical messengers of mind and
mood called neurotransmitters. As they travel around your brain and nervous
system, neurotransmitters help determine how you feel.

Here's the important part: We can influence our brain function by supplying the right nutrients to make our brain cells and neurotransmitters work at their peak.

There are hundreds of neurotransmitters. These are the main players:

GABA (gamma-aminobutyric acid) is the "cool" neurotransmitter, relaxing you and calming you down during periods of stress.

Adrenaline (also called *epinephrine*), made in the adrenal glands, is the "motivator," stimulating you and helping you respond to stress.

Dopamine and **noradrenaline** (also called *norepinephrine*) are the "feel-good" neurotransmitters, making you feel energized and in control.

Endorphins promote that blissful feeling, giving you a sense of euphoria.

Acetylcholine works on memory and concentration.

Serotonin is the "happy" and calming neurotransmitter, improving your mood and helping you to sleep well.

Melatonin helps to keep you in tune with the cycles of nature by responding to seasonal shifts and regulating your inner clock for day and night. It affects your ability to sleep soundly and to dream.

When these neurotransmitters are out of balance, you may feel depressed, anxious, stressed and unmotivated—or any other mental problem that you can imagine. On the other hand, with balanced neurotransmitters you are calm and happy and can think clearly. You are able to handle all the challenges that life throws at you, and enjoy all the wonders as well.

THE FOOD CONNECTION

"You are what you eat."
—R. J. CRUMBE

The protein we eat is broken down by digestive processes into its component amino acids. For brain function, the most important amino acids are tryptophan, tyrosine, GABA, glutamine and taurine. They are turned into neurotransmitters with the help of cofactors, or chemical helpers: vitamins B_3, B_6, B_{12}, C, and folic acid (folate), and the minerals zinc and magnesium. In addition, you need the essential fatty acids that make up about 60% of each brain cell.

Then there's glucose (blood sugar) required for fuel. Amazingly, that little three-pound organ, your brain, can use up to half of the body's glucose at any one time. That's why we feel so good when we have a sugar high—it goes right to our brain, where it's burned for fuel! The same is true of processed foods, alcohol, and caffeine. You'll get a quick high, but in a short time, it's used up and your body wants more. Stay on that sugar roller coaster and eventually you'll start suffering blood sugar dips and increasing mood swings. (See Chapter 13 for more information on blood sugar imbalances.)

In addition to foods, certain medications, including antihistamines, tranquilizers, sleeping pills, narcotics and recreational drugs can affect your brain chemistry.

DEPRESSION AND ANXIETY

We need sufficient amounts of the key neurotransmitters to stay centered, calm, and happy. In depression, there is a lack of mood-stabilizing serotonin and noradrenaline as well as dopamine, the brain chemicals associated with motivation and pleasure and derived from tyrosine.

To make serotonin, your brain needs enough of the essential amino acid tryptophan, found in protein-containing foods like turkey, chicken, cottage cheese, avocados, bananas, and wheat germ. Supplementation with the amino acid 5-hydroxytryptophan can also help your brain manufacture more serotonin.

Noradrenaline deficiency often results in cravings for stimulation from sugar, coffee, stress, and alcohol. Supplementation with the amino acids tyrosine and phenylalanine can convert to dopamine, which helps your brain manufacture more noradrenaline.

With anxiety, there is a deficiency in the neurotransmitter GABA, the brain's "anti-stimulant." Formed from the amino acids glutamine, GABA, and taurine, low GABA means high anxiety.

Besides your food intake, there are dozens of reasons why your neurotransmitters may become depleted; among them are diabetes, liver disease, autoimmune disease, heart disease, high blood pressure, cancer, blood pressure–lowering medications, birth control pills, tranquilizers, antidepressants and stimulants. Depression and anxiety can also be caused by blood sugar imbalances, sex hormone imbalances, food and chemical sensitivities, toxins and candida, so it might be helpful for you to read those sections of this book as well.

We all get the blues from time to time in response to life events. Occasional bouts of sadness help us appreciate the good times. Most of us bounce back within a day or two or maybe even a week or two. But sometimes we get "stuck" in that feeling of being unable to cope, and that leads to depression.

SYMPTOMS OF DEPRESSION

- Profound, persistent sadness
- Profound, persistent irritability
- Unexplained crying
- Loss of self-esteem
- Feelings of hopelessness, helplessness, pessimism, worthlessness, guilt, and emptiness
- Dwelling on the past, particularly on errors you think you've made
- Changes in sleeping patterns
- Changes in eating habits
- Unexplained weight gain or loss
- Restlessness
- Fatigue
- A slowdown in physical movements
- Inability to concentrate
- Memory difficulties
- Difficulty making decisions
- Loss of interest in usually pleasurable activities
- Loss of interest in sex
- Social withdrawal
- Unexplained headaches, stomach upset, or other physical problems that are not helped with a standard treatment
- Thoughts of suicide or death

SYMPTOMS OF ANXIETY

- Abdominal discomfort
- Diarrhea
- Dry mouth
- Rapid heartbeat or palpitations
- Tightness or pain in chest
- Shortness of breath
- Frequent urination
- Difficulty swallowing
- Insomnia
- Irritability or anger
- Inability to concentrate
- Fear you're losing control of your actions

Here are examples of both types of responses:

My patient Stacey told me she was "a wreck" after her boyfriend of three years announced that he wanted his freedom. However, with the help of some brief counseling and the support of her friends, she soon got through her feelings of loss and began dating again.

Her friend Janet, on the other hand, found herself in similar circumstances, with very different results. When Janet's relationship ended, she was in tears for months. She withdrew from friends and family, was unable to sleep, began to perform poorly at work, and felt like a total failure. Her response seemed somewhat extreme, and she was on a downward spiral, heading toward a severe clinical depression.

Why were their responses so different? First check out the "Symptoms of Depression." If you or anyone you know have more than three of these, please seek professional help. There is no shame in having this condition, and the help you get can be life-saving.

Severe, clinically recognizable depression affects one in five people at some time in their lives. Some of the symptoms of depression applied to Janet. They may occur one at a time or in combination. They generally come upon you gradually, but can be brought on by a crisis as in Janet's case. She also felt nervous and worried, verging on panic. These are all signs of anxiety, which occurs when your brain begins sending messages to your body to prepare for the "fight-or-flight" response, as you can see on the "Symptoms of Anxiety" list.

Most of us are able to take adversity in stride, yet clearly some people are more resilient than others, depending on genetics, personal history, and lifestyle. Are there ways to handle the difficult times?

In a word, "yes."

Let's look at the ways depression and anxiety can be handled, with the pros and cons of each approach. Most importantly: If you or someone you know is severely depressed, please contact a health professional for help.

Traditional Medical Treatment

Millions of people are taking prescription drugs for depression and anxiety. If you think they're safe and effective, I have news for you: They're not. These drugs are effective in only about 50% of the cases, and the majority of people taking them suffer a variety of side effects as well, some fairly serious. Here are a few of the most commonly used prescription drugs and their side effects:

Selective serotonin reuptake inhibitors, also called SSRIs (Prozac, Paxil, Zoloft, Luvox, Celexa): These enormously popular drugs block the re-absorption of "feel-good" serotonin, thereby making more serotonin available and elevating mood. Unfortunately, they also compromise libido and sexual performance in men and women, cause "flat" moods or a lack of emotional highs and lows and can bring on other side effects including nausea, nervousness, insomnia, headache, tremors, anxiety, drowsiness, dry mouth, excessive sweating and diarrhea. SSRIs can also have serious long-term withdrawal effects.

Tricyclic antidepressants (Elavil, Endep, Tofranil, Pertofane, Norpramin, Sinequan): These popular drugs work in various ways to affect the actions of noradrenaline and serotonin. They can cause dizziness, drowsiness, heart palpitations, dry mouth, blurred vision, confusion, weight gain, sweating, rashes, nausea, constipation or diarrhea, difficulty urinating, sexual dysfunction, nightmares and anxiety.

Monoamine oxidase inhibitors, also called MAOIs (Nardil, Parnate, Manerix):

These work by inhibiting or reducing the levels of monoamine oxidase, or MAO. This in turn increases the levels of "feel-good" brain chemicals such as serotonin, norepinephrine, and dopamine by preventing their breakdown in the brain. They can cause dangerously high blood pressure if taken with decongestants, antihistamines or foods containing tyramine, such as cheese or red wine.

Benzodiazepines (Valium, Xanax, Klonopin, Restoril, Ativan): These tranquilizers slow down the central nervous system to reduce anxiety. They can cause drowsiness, irregular heartbeat, memory loss, disorientation, low blood pressure and muscle weakness. Benzodiazepines are almost certainly addictive when taken for a long period of time and cause withdrawal symptoms if stopped suddenly.

There are a few other types of antidepressant and anti-anxiety medications that don't fit into the categories we mentioned, including Wellbutrin, Effexor, and Cymbalta.

As bad as the side effects of these medications might seem, there is a place for them, particularly in lower doses than are generally prescribed. In his groundbreaking book *Over Dose* (Tarcher, 2004), Dr. Jay Cohen explains how the drug companies recommend far higher doses than are generally necessary. For example, the optimal dose for Prozac was found to be one-half to one-fourth the usual recommended dose. Moreover, women require lower doses than men do, though that is seldom taken into consideration. In any case, synthetic pharmaceutical medications should be reserved for those times when their benefits clearly outweigh their downsides.

When you want to combine natural products with prescription medication, do so under a doctor's supervision to ensure that there are no negative interactions.

Talk Therapy

There are various types of psychotherapy or "talk" therapy, which can be very helpful in dealing with depression. In my practice, I prefer to use the more rapid therapies such as EMDR (Eye Movement Desensitization and Reprocessing), guided imagery or Voice Dialogue (developed by Drs. Hal and Sidra

Stone, www.delos-inc.com). I have found that therapy works much better once brain chemistry is balanced.

Changes in Diet

Often, successful treatment of depression and anxiety can be as simple as treating blood sugar imbalances (see Chapter 13). Low blood sugar can cause mood swings and anxiety, so we recommend that you eat small, frequent meals to prevent blood sugar swings. In addition: Avoid alcohol, which is a depressant. It's the last thing you need when you're feeling low. And ditch the caffeine because it can leave you feeling drained and jittery.

Increase your intake of essential fatty acids in the form of fatty fish like salmon and tuna or in flaxseed oil to give your body the building material for optimal neurotransmitter production. Eat sufficient protein in the form of fish, poultry, meat or soy (tofu) to provide the raw materials to make neurotransmitters.

Natural Approaches to Depression and Anxiety

Although prescription drugs can sometimes be useful, over my years of practice, I've learned that natural supplements should be the first line of treatment. They are gentle and safe. Rather than simply dealing with the symptoms, they actually correct the underlying imbalances.

Here is a list of supplements that I have successfully used in my own practice, all backed by research. Also remember to have a look at the de-stress supplements listed on pages 114–117.

St. John's wort (*hypericum perforatum*): Dozens of studies have proven St. John's wort's ability to relieve, and even eliminate, mild to moderate depression. It is shown to be effective in 60 to 80% of people who take it. It compares well with to the prescription antidepressants, without their side effects. It may even boost sex drive! There are more advantages to taking St. John's wort: It's not addictive, it doesn't interact negatively with alcohol, it doesn't cause withdrawal symptoms if you stop taking it, it doesn't make you sleepy in the daytime, but it does help you sleep at night. While I've had several patients that needed 2–3 weeks to have it work fully, St. John's wort often begins working within days, unlike the SSRIs that take weeks to be fully effective.

Animal studies show St. John's wort, like the SSRI antidepressants, enhances serotonin, and likely, dopamine and noradrenaline as well.

Cautions: May cause allergic reactions, rashes, gastrointestinal upset or sun sensitivity in some people. Can cause anxiety or insomnia if taken too close to bedtime. It can reduce the potency of protease inhibitors (taken as a treatment for AIDS) or cyclosporine (an immunosuppressant taken by organ transplant patients), digoxin (heart medication) or even birth control pills. If combined with an SSRI or 5-HTP, there's a very slight possibility of serotonin syndrome consisting of nausea, sweating, headache and a rise in temperature and blood pressure. If that occurs, stop the St. John's wort and seek medical help.

Dosage: Start with one or two capsules of a 300 mg of an extract with 0.3% hypericin, three times daily, for a total of 900 mg a day. You can also take your entire dose in the morning, since the herb is quite long-acting.

5-HTP (5-hydroxytryptophan): Derived from tryptophan, the "happy" and calming neurotransmitter, 5-HTP is converted into serotonin, causing you to feel relaxed, in a good mood and able to fall asleep and stay asleep. Another great benefit of 5-HTP: It suppresses appetite. It may be preferable to tryptophan because 5-HTP enters the brain more easily and it can be taken with food and other supplements, including amino acids, with no problem. 5-HTP also suppresses appetite and helps in migraine prevention.

Cautions: In rare cases at very high doses, 5-HTP can cause nausea, anxiety and agitation. For some sensitive individuals it can cause anxiety at normal levels as well. Do not take 5-HTP with SSRIs except under medical guidance. While generally safe to combine, there is a risk of serotonin syndrome—nausea, sweating, headache and a rise in blood pressure. If that occurs, stop the 5-HTP.

Dosage: Take 50–100 mg two to three times daily for daytime usage. To promote sleep, 50–200 mg one hour before bedtime. Be sure to take 25 mg of vitamin B_6 to help convert the 5-HTP to serotonin. It can be part of your daily multivitamin formula. To prevent migraines, take 100–300 mg daily.

SAM-e (s-adenosyl-methionine) or TMG (trimethylglycine): Both act as natural mood enhancers by enhancing neurotransmitter activity. TMG, which is much less expensive, provides the raw material from which your body manufactures SAM-e.

Cautions: High doses may lead to irritability, anxiety, insomnia, nausea or vomiting. In people with bipolar disorder, SAM-e (like any antidepressant) may trigger a manic episode, so such individuals should be monitored carefully. Do not take SAM-e and TMG if you are taking prescription antidepressants, unless you're under a doctor's supervision.

Dosage: SAM-e: take 200 mg once or twice daily, between meals, increasing gradually to a maximum of 1,600 mg a day, if needed. Generally, 400–800 mg a day will do. TMG: take 500–1,000 mg once or twice daily.

DL-phenylalanine and L- tyrosine, simply called phenylalanine and tyrosine: These are *the* supplements to help you get a real energy boost, lift your mood, relieve pain and control appetite. DL-phenylalanine (DLPA) converts to tyrosine, which help your body make dopamine, noradrenaline and finally, adrenaline.

Cautions: You could get too much stimulation, causing anxiety, high blood pressure or insomnia. These shouldn't be taken by people with phenylketonuria or melanoma, or by pregnant or nursing women. Use caution with a history of bipolar illness, since they act as antidepressants and can (rarely) induce mania.

Dosage: Take 500–1,000 mg of DLPA and 100–1,000 mg of tyrosine twice daily on an empty stomach. Do not take close to bedtime. Avoid proteins for two hours before or after, if possible, to prevent interference with absorption.

Rhodiola (*rhodiola rosea*): Rhodiola is an *adaptogenic herb,* meaning that it helps to regulate your system in response to stress. Russian research shows that rhodiola can enhance your body's production of serotonin, dopamine and norepinephrine, enabling it to both lift your mood and calm your nerves. It helps to increase both energy and mental performance, and even has been shown to encourage weight loss.

Cautions: There are no known side effects.

Dosage: Use 100–300 mg of a standardized product.

For the anxiety that often accompanies depression, see the remedies for stress

Now, back to Janet. She responded well to high doses of B vitamins and 3 grams daily of essential fatty acids, plus a high-potency multivitamin and a "beat-the-blues" cocktail of St. John's wort, 5-HTP, and tyrosine. Three months later, she bounced into my office, eager to share confidences about the new love in her life—and her renewed interest in sex and romance!

Once her equilibrium was established, over the next three months she gradually decreased the tyrosine and B vitamins, then dropped the 5-HTP, and finally went down to one dose of St. John's wort daily. She remained on the multi vitamin and fish oil. She had also discovered marathon running, and that did a lot to boost her mood, as research confirms. Of course, the new boyfriend was also a great mood lifter.

Coming Off Prescription Medications

If you are taking anti-anxiety drugs or antidepressants, you have a lot of company. There are certainly withdrawal effects from benzodiazepines and there may be similar effects from SSRIs. If you choose to stop taking these medications, you must do so under medical supervision. Abrupt withdrawal from benzodiazepines can cause seizures or even death.

It takes months to get off these drugs successfully. The program should be tailored to the individual's needs and carefully monitored by a medical professional. Natural remedies such as kava and valerian can shorten the gradual program of withdrawal from benzodiazepines.

If you want to end dependency on these drugs, read the chapter on addiction in my book, *Natural Highs,* and share it with your doctor. In most situations, you can combine natural products with medication. Do so under a doctor's supervision to ensure that there are no negative interactions.

MEMORY LOSS AND LACK OF CONCENTRATION

It's happened to all of us: fuzzy thinking, daydreaming, inability to concentrate, a slow mind and the struggle to connect names with faces or recall schedules and phone numbers.

We often will turn to stimulants like sugar and coffee in a vain effort to jump-start our minds.

Declining mental function, which often starts when we reach our forties, is not inevitable. We've got good news for you: You can get your mind in gear again and make it work better than ever.

Some simple interventions can go a long way. Mira brought her 75-year-old mother, Dora, to see me. Her memory had become so bad that Mira was afraid to leave her alone in her nearby apartment. Dora was forgetful, getting lost in the neighborhood and appeared depressed. Her doctor wanted to prescribe antidepressants, but Mira wasn't convinced. She knew how much help she herself had found through natural means.

TEST YOUR MEMORY

Here's a questionnaire to help you determine how good (or bad) your memory is. Answer "yes" or "no" to each question.

1. Is your memory deteriorating?   _____

2. Do you find it hard to concentrate?   _____

3. Do you often get confused?   _____

4. Do you sometimes forget the name of someone you know quite well? _____

5. Do you often find you can remember things from the past but forget what you did yesterday?   _____

6. Do you ever forget what day of the week it is?   _____

7. Do your friends and family think you're more forgetful than you once were?   _____

8. Do you find it hard to add numbers without writing them down?   _____

9. Do you often misplace your keys?   _____

10. Do you frequently repeat yourself?   _____

11. Do you sometimes forget the point you were trying to make?   _____

12. Does it take you longer to learn things than it once did?   _____

If you answered "yes" to fewer than four questions, you may not have a major problem with your memory, but you'll find that natural mind and memory boosters will sharpen your memory even more. If you answered "yes" to five to eight questions, your memory definitely needs a boost. Read on. If you answered "yes" to nine questions or more, you are experiencing significant memory decline. In addition to following the Vibrant Health Plan diet and supplement recommendations, see a natural health practitioner who can help you identify other causes of memory decline, such as a hormone imbalance or stress, especially if you scored high on the life stress questionnaire in Chapter 9.

Mental decline can be due to disease of the blood vessels (vascular disease; hypertension) or to neurotoxins. The circulatory problems are addressed with a multi-pronged approach, beginning with the Vibrant Health Plan. Circulatory problems will likely respond to chelation therapy, given intravenously or orally, which uses a chelating or "grabbing" agent to clear the calcium deposits from the arterial walls. You can find details on chelation therapy at www.acam.org. For dealing with toxins, see Chapter 15.

Here's what you can do for prevention. First of all, it's a "use it or lose it" situation. The more you "exercise" your brain, the better it will work. Whether you're 20 or 60, the time to act is *now.* You must maintain a proper diet, exercise, reduce stress levels, get rid of toxins in the brain, and take nutrients that boost mental function.

One quick way to get a handle on memory loss is to reduce stress. Researchers at Stanford University have found that the communication system among brain cells begins to shrivel up after just two weeks of exposure to stress-induced high cortisol levels. (See Chapter 9 on stress imbalances.) The great news is that managing stress can reverse the effect.

Be sure you're getting plenty of antioxidants in your diet, including foods containing large amounts of vitamins A, C, and E, selenium and zinc. These are needed to neutralize free radicals, which are toxic molecules formed by our normal metabolism as well as toxins we take into our bodies from our environment.

Our trillions of brain cells are made of 60 to 70% fats or lipids, and we need essential fatty acids (EFAs) to provide the appropriate raw materials. So include plenty of "brain food" in the form of fatty fish (salmon, mackerel, tuna), flaxseeds and oils made from seeds and nuts. Avoid the bad fats: trans-fatty acids and saturated fats.

Standard Medical Treatment

Aricept (donepezil) has been shown to slow the progression of Alzheimer's disease only minimally if at all. Side effects include loss of appetite, vomiting, muscle cramps, fatigue and diarrhea.

Natural Approaches

Natural treatments provide the materials needed to make brain cells and enhance neurotransmitter production and activity. Find more details, including recommended doses and cautions, in the Appendix.

Acetyl-L-Carnitine: This amino acid improves mood and mental performance. It is fuel for the brain and helps make the memory neurotransmitter acetylcholine. It also acts as an antioxidant for the brain and nervous system.
Cautions: Not recommended for people with diabetes, liver or kidney disease.
Dosage: Take 250–1,500 mg daily, between meals.

Choline: This is part of the structure of neuronal membranes and one of the building blocks of acetylcholine, neurotransmitter that is key to improving memory and mental alertness, and declines with age. Choline and its derivatives will help you feel more alert, clear-headed and improves memory and concentration. It's even recommended to help improve the brain development of your baby while you're pregnant.
Cautions: Choline has no cautions, except it can make you smell fishy (sorry). However, there are variations that don't do that.
Dosage: (Daily) 5–10 g (approximately 1 tablespoon) of lecithin, *or* 2.5–5 g (a heaping tablespoon) of hi-phosphatidylcholine lecithin, *or* 1–2 g of phosphatidyl choline, 500–1,000 mg of citicholine and 500–1,500 mg of alpha-GPC (my preference).

Dimethylaminoethanol (DMAE): DMAE increases alertness, improves concentration, reduces anxiety, improves learning and attention span and normalizes brain-wave patterns. DMAE is the building block for acetylcholine that crosses easily into the brain.
Cautions: Too much DMAE can be over stimulating, so if you experience insomnia, lower the dose.
Dosage: Take 100–300 mg daily in the morning or at midday. Do not take in the evening.

Ginkgo Biloba: This herbal extract from the leaf of the ancient ginkgo tree increases circulation to the brain and has been shown to increase serotonin levels in the elderly. Research shows that it not only prevents the progression of Alzheimer's disease, but can enhance mood, memory, concentration, mental performance and energy in younger people as well.

Cautions: Because ginkgo has a mild blood-thinning effect, do not combine it with anticoagulant drugs like Coumadin, heparin or aspirin.

Dosage: 120 mg a day of extract standardized to 24 to 28% ginkgo flavonglycosides.

Experiment with various combinations of these remedies, adding in one at a time and seeing how you respond. They can be safely combined as I do in my practice. For more details see *Natural Highs*.

Back to Dora, who sat listless and withdrawn next to her daughter Mira. With Dora's permission, I gave her an injection of B vitamins, predominantly B_{12} and folic acid. This had an almost immediate effect on her demeanor and energy. She perked up and began recounting times in the past when her family doctor had given her "energy shots" of B_{12}. After giving her a prescription for some lab work, I drew up a list of supplements for her to take in addition to the usual program (you know what it is by now!): vitamin B_{12} to take under her tongue daily (for better absorption), ginkgo, phosphatidylcholine and phosphatidylserine and a few other supplements in a combined formula for ease of use.

Within eight weeks, Dora had regained many of her faculties. A miracle? Yes and no. Her vitamin B_{12} deficiency, common in the elderly who often absorb it poorly, was interfering with her neurotransmitter production. The ginkgo helped restore brain blood flow, getting more oxygen to her brain. Her new-found alertness and energy inspired her to take daily walks in the park which helped even further. Fresh air, sunlight, exercise, and nature all have healing effects on the brain and body.

Brain chemistry imbalances can be devastating, but the recovery can be quick and sustained.

Natural Approaches for Migraines

Coenzyme Q_{10}: CoQ_{10} has been show to prevent migraines in a large number of patients. It has many benefits, including enhancing energy and well-being. CoQ_{10} is the body's energy catalyst, the beginning point of a chain of chemical reactions that create the energy or ATP your cells need to function at an optimal level. It works within the mitochondria, the energy generators in every cell of the body. It's also a powerful antioxidant that gobbles up disease-causing free radicals and enhances blood glucose, heart, kidney and liver function. Adding quercetin to CoQ_{10} can make it even more effective as a migraine treatment.

Cautions: CoQ_{10} may cause mild gastrointestinal upset. Taking it late in the day can cause insomnia.

Dosage: The usual dosage of CoQ_{10} is 1 mg per pound of body weight, so if you weigh 150 pounds, you'll need 150 mg of CoQ_{10}. If you take the more absorbable softgels, you'll need only about two-thirds of that dosage, which can save you money, since CoQ_{10} is a little pricey.

Feverfew: One of the most effective herbs for migraine prevention is feverfew. It regulates serotonin secretion, although it may take up three months to be fully effective.

Cautions: May decrease blood clotting ability, so it should not be taken with anticoagulant drugs. Should not be used by pregnant women because it can cause uterine contractions.

Dosage: 250 mg taken every morning. Look for a preparation standardized to contain 4% parthenolide.

Magnesium: Half of all migraine sufferers are low in magnesium, which has a direct effect on serotonin balance. Intravenous magnesium administered in a doctor's office can stop a migraine in progress.

Cautions: May cause diarrhea and has been rarely associated with blood sugar drops.

Dosage: 500–1,000 mg daily of chelated form (aspartate, glycinate, citrate) for prevention.

Riboflavin: Vitamin B-2 or riboflavin has been shown to improve cell communication in the brain. With long term use, B-2 helped relieve frequency of attacks in 68% of those who took it. There are excellent combination supplements that, based on clinical research, provide the amounts of feverfew, magnesium and riboflavin that are effective in preventing migraines,.

Cautions: None.

Dosage: 200–400 mg daily.

5-HTP: *See depression.*

Acupuncture

The ancient Chinese therapy is an effective way of balancing serotonin production and has been shown in studies to reduce migraine severity by nearly 40%.

Experiment with various combinations of these remedies, adding in one at a time and seeing how you respond. They can be safely combined as I do in my practice.

Brain chemistry imbalances can be devastating, but the recovery can be exciting and fast with the right combination of supplements, diet and mind-body approaches.

CONCLUSION

The brain is a remarkable organ. Weighing in at a mere three pounds, it can be the abode of fear, anxiety, deep depression and severe physical pain. It also has the capacity to hold countless memories and allows us to experience the beauty of music, the ecstasy of love, the thrills of sex and the bliss of inner peace. Your new understanding of how the brain works will help you to decrease the negative experiences and enhance the positive ones.

11

SEX HORMONES: FROM PMS TO MENOPAUSE

Jamie, a 27-year-old eighth-grade teacher, complained that her hormonal swings and those of her pubescent students were a match made in hell. "A week before my period, I become a different person. I eat everything in sight, and I pick on my kids mercilessly. Then I stress because I am acting like such a terror. I hate this Jekyll and Hyde thing that I'm doing, or, in fact, it's doing me!"

Then there's Alicia. At 51, she was clearly in the throes of menopause. I could see the sheen of sweat on her forehead as she sat in my air-conditioned office, and I recognized the discomfort of the extra pounds she was carrying. "My husband must be a saint, coping with my cranky moods, my tears and the sweat-soaked bedsheets," she said, shaking her head in resignation.

As women, we all know the feelings associated with hormone swings, whether during menstrual cycles or when hormone production begins to decline with age, a period known as "perimenopause," en route to menopause.

Women's hormonal structure, indeed our very DNA structure, makes us the more complex sex. There's no question: Throughout our lives we labor harder in the physical, mental, and emotional sense. Our reward is that we are susceptible to far fewer genetic diseases and we live an average of seven years longer than men do.

Our mothers once called them "women's problems." Now we know that these mood swings and physical changes, from PMS to menopause, are all part of a delicate balance among our various hormones.

So, what are hormones, anyway? They are chemical messengers secreted by any one of the body's endocrine (ductless) glands: the thyroid (thyroid hormone), parathyroid (parathormone), ovaries (estrogen, progesterone), testes (testosterone), adrenals (adrenaline, cortisol, DHEA) and pancreas (insulin). They travel through the bloodstream, telling various systems what to do. Besides reproductive functions, hormones affect virtually every body system from digestion to metabolism to hair growth.

In this chapter, we'll be dealing with the main female sex hormones estrogen and progesterone, and we'll see what happens when they get out of balance at various stages of life.

THE HORMONAL SYMPHONY

Each woman is an individual. Your hormonal profile is as unique as your fingerprint. The only way you can know your true hormone status is by testing levels of the major hormones.

Estrogen. We've all heard of estrogen, but most of us may not realize that there are three forms of estrogen: estrone, estradiol and estriol. Proper estrogen balances enhance sleep, mood, mental sharpness and memory, digestion, sex drive, skin tone, and brain chemicals such as the "feel-good" hormones serotonin and endorphins. European research indicates that estriol may also protect against cancer. Estrogen may also protect you against osteoporosis, heart disease, Alzheimer's disease, colon cancer, urinary incontinence and tooth decay. We are referring here to natural estrogens, either those made by your body or manufactured *bioidentical hormones* that are the same in structure.

Progesterone. This hormone is produced by your ovaries after ovulation, during the second half of your menstrual cycle. It is necessary for fertility, for maintaining pregnancy, and to address a host of perimenopausal and menopausal symptoms. Progesterone is a mood enhancer. It has a calming effect, regulates fluid balance in your body to prevent bloating, increases energy and sex drive, decreases the risk of cancer of the endometrium (the lining of the uterus), stabilizes blood sugar, thyroid function, and mineral balance, and may help protect against breast cancer, fibrocystic breasts, and osteoporosis.

Testosterone. We can hear you now: That's a *male* hormone! True, and women have it, too. It is the hormone of desire in both sexes. Natural testosterone levels diminish after menopause, although your ovaries and adrenal glands continue to produce small amounts. Testosterone helps with tissue growth and stimulates blood flow. It can help relieve menopausal symptoms like depression, bone loss, and diminished sex drive. It's important not to overdo the testosterone, because an overdose can cause acne, oily skin, facial hair growth and aggressive behavior. In fact, you might notice yourself being uncharacteristically impatient in traffic or easy to anger when someone cuts you off. One of my patients, a normally sweet, well-mannered teacher, realized that her testosterone dose was too high when the following happened: while trying to enter a dance club one evening with her girlfriends, she got into an argument with the doorman, and was nearly arrested for disorderly conduct!

DHEA. The tongue-twister hormone dehydroepiandrosterone has been called the "fountain of youth" hormone. Manufactured by the adrenal glands rather than the ovaries, its levels decline as we age. Having enough DHEA enhances your immune function, possibly lowers cholesterol, enhances sex drive and mood, and improves insulin function. It helps to lower levels of the stress hormone cortisol. Too much DHEA can have the same effect as too much testosterone, plus irritability and insomnia. It may also contribute to breast cancer if your body converts it to the "bad" estrogen. More on that later.

Pregenenolone. The hormone produced by the adrenal glands is the "mother" or source of all hormones. It is the building block from which all hormones in your body are created. At the age of 50, your pregenenolone levels are half what they were when you were 25. An anti-aging supplement, it helps improve memory and hormone levels, connective tissue and degenerative disorders; nerve cell damage; and the ravages of stress. It also enhances the benefits of DHEA.

SHBG (sex hormone binding globulin). Sometimes called the "chaperone" of estrogen, SHBG accompanies estrogen as it moves through your bloodstream. When the estrogen levels in your bloodstream are too high, your liver recognizes the imbalance and pumps out extra SHBG to keep the estrogen levels under control, releasing more as needed.

This complex interplay of hormones becomes problematic for women as we age because SHBG binds to all types of hormones, including thyroid, human growth hormone and testosterone, making them unavailable for use. Oral contraceptives also increase the level of SHBG, interfering with hormone availability throughout the body. This would explain the lack of libido in many women on brith control pills: Testosterone, the 'sexy" hormones, is bound and thus less available where it's needed.

PREMENSTRUAL SYNDROME (PMS)

Let's get back to Jamie, our schoolteacher, who describes herself as a "terror" before her period, picking on her students, overeating, and feeling quite out of control.

To begin with, it's important to understand the basic phases of the menstrual cycle.

Most of us have a cycle of 24 to 35 days. The average cycle is about 28 days, but our exposure to environmental and plant estrogens may be shortening our cycles, laying the groundwork for hormonal and fertility problems.

Day 1 is the day bleeding begins. Most women's periods last two to seven days, and they lose about four tablespoons of blood. This is called the menstrual phase.

The time between the end of your period and ovulation is a time of increasing estrogen production. It's called the follicular phase, when the egg is maturing and preparing to be fertilized.

Ovulation, the release of the egg from the ovaries, takes place about midcycle, and your ovaries begin to produce progesterone at that time. If the egg is fertilized, you are pregnant and the cycle won't resume until after the baby is born.

About two weeks after ovulation, if the egg is not fertilized, your uterus will shed its lining along with the unfertilized egg. This is when estrogen and progesterone drop totheir lowest point, which may trigger PMS symptoms. Probably most of us have experienced PMS like Jamie's from time to time. The cramps, headaches, backaches and general crankiness just before your period begins are not only an annoyance, these symptoms can become so severe that they interfere with your relationships and your work.

PMS Symptoms

• Psychological: tension, irritability, fatigue, panic, phobia

- Breasts: tender, swollen

- Nervous system: migraine, headaches, fainting, dizziness, seizures

- Skin: acne, herpes, hives, boils

- Muscles and joints: backache, joint pain, bloating

- Gastrointestinal system: food cravings, bloating, gas

- Urinary: bladder infections

- Water retention: increased weight, tight-fitting rings

Conventional Medical Treatment

There are few medical ways of treating PMS. Many doctors believe it is strictly an emotional disorder. They will often prescribe antidepressants called SSRIs (selective serotonin reuptake inhibitors such as Prozac, Zoloft, Paxil, Celexa or Lexapro) for premenstrual depression or anxiety. Some doctors will recommend over-the-counter nonsteroidal anti-inflammatory drugs (NSAIDs) like ibuprofen or non-NSAIDs such as acetaminophen.

Check your hormones, including thyroid and progesterone levels. This can be done with a saliva test, best taken at intervals throughout the month in order to track the pattern.

Diet and Lifestyle

Eat fewer animal products and add raw broccoli and other cruciferous veggies to your salads. Reduce or eliminate caffeine, alcohol, nicotine and sugar. Reduce or eliminate high-fat dairy products. Eliminate as much processed food as possible. Reduce salt intake. Eat small regular meals.

Yoga and meditation are helpful for PMS sufferers because they work on the nervous system and help balance hormones.

Natural Supplements

Here are supplements that I find most useful. Find more details, including recommended doses and cautions, in the Appendix.

Magnesium: This essential mineral is involved in more than 300 body processes, including countering the fluid retention that so many women experience before their periods. It's also responsible for helping your body assimilate calcium and vitamin D (see next paragraph). Magnesium is also an important for migraine prevention and relief. If you crave chocolate just before your period, you may actually be craving the magnesium in chocolate.

Cautions: Excessive magnesium acts as a laxative so take it to "bowel tolerance". Use chelated forms such as magnesium aspartate, glycinate or citrate which is absorbed and utilized more efficiently than the more common (and less expensive) magnesium oxide

Dosage: Take 200–400 mg up to three times daily. Take the last dose at bedtime. To increase absorption, be sure to get 30–50 mg of vitamin B_6, best in a B-complex supplement.

Calcium and vitamin D: We all know how important these minerals are for strong bones and teeth, but most of us aren't aware how important calcium is for hormone regulation. Estrogen also regulates calcium metabolism and through a complex series of events, it triggers fluctuations all the way through the menstrual cycle. Research also suggests that calcium and vitamin D therapy is helpful in treating hormonally related migraines.

Cautions: None at this dosage.

Dosage: Be sure you're getting at least 1,200–1,500 mg of calcium a day and a minimum of 1,000 IU of vitamin D, which is essential for the absorption of calcium. You'll also need 3 mg of boron daily. Balance it with magnesium for optimum utilization by the body. You'll find many combination products that contain the precise mixture you need. Take the last dose at bedtime.

Gamma-Linoleic Acid: GLA, an essential omega-6 fatty acid, is found in evening primrose, borage seed and black currant oils that, among many other benefits, help relieve depression and irritability, breast tenderness and fluid retention linked with PMS.

Cautions: None at this dosage.

Dosage: Take 900 mg twice daily.

Chasteberry (*vitex agnus castus*): Also known as Vitex, this herb effects the production of luteinizing hormones, influencing progesterone levels in the last phase of the menstrual cycle, just before your period. This reduces mood swings, headaches and breast tenderness.

Cautions: Do not use chasteberry if you might become pregnant or if you are taking hormone therapies of any kind (including thyroid medication) or anti-depressants.

Dosage: 20–120 mg per day in capsule form or 40 drops of liquid extract.

Consider taking these supplements in addition to your high-potency multi-vitamin: vitamin B complex (50 mg a day), zinc (up to 50 mg daily), and chromium (up to 400 mcg daily).

You may also consider adding mixed bioflavonoids (500 mg twice a day) and melatonin (1 mg at bedtime for several days mid-cycle and several days before your period).

For depression, add these one at a time and see what works best for you:

- Extra chromium (200 mcg twice a day)

- 5-HTP (50–100 mg twice a day, or take the whole dose at bedtime if it makes you drowsy).

- St. John's wort (300 mg three times a day standardized to 0.3% hypericin. You can take the whole dose at once with breakfast, too).

- Tyrosine (500–1,000 mg once or twice daily (but not after 3 PM or so since it's stimulating, the week before your period and during your period if needed).

For breast tenderness, take indole-3-carbinol (200 mg twice a day). It helps metabolize excess estrogen and restore hormonal balance (see details below).

For natural hormone therapy, take natural progesterone cream (up to 30 mg daily) for one week prior to your period. This is not yam cream. While it may have some positive effects, to raise progesterone you need the bio-identical product. Prescription doses are higher. I generally prescribe a 10% cream or 100 mg per gram, which can be used in tiny dabs of up to one gram daily to ease symptoms. Since progesterone tends to be calming, it is best taken at bed-time. However, you can choose your preferred time, based on your body's response.

Jamie watched her diet, eliminated the sweet and salty foods she had been craving and added my PMS Balance formula that contains vitamin B_6, borage oil and chasteberry among other herbal ingredients (available at www.drcass. com). In addition, she took magnesium and her multi. Within two months she was a changed woman. "Voilà! The world is so much better, and I'm so much nicer to be around. I even like myself more," she joked.

ESTROGEN DOMINANCE

We are currently seeing an increase in many female-hormone-related conditions, from premature puberty (as young as two years of age!), to increased incidence of PMS, infertility, endometriosis, severe menopausal symptoms and breast and other female cancers. Environmental toxins such as dioxin (from pesticides and plastics) are fake estrogens, or "xenoestrogens," attaching to the estrogen receptors and creating a perceived estrogen excess in the body. This affects the estrogen to progesterone ratio, which is the basis for good hormonal regulation. A relative deficiency of progesterone then occurs and hormonal havoc ensues. D. Lindsey Berkson's excellent book *Hormone Deception* (McGraw-Hill, 2001) goes into depth about this growing problem and some of its solutions. You will find more on toxins in Chapter 15.

Estrogen dominance also occurs during perimenopause, during "anovulatory" cycles, when an egg fails to be released. Because there is no signal from the egg to the ovary to release progesterone, there remains only unopposed estrogen, which causes the problems we're describing.

A related issue is the creation of too much "bad" (2-hydroxy-estrogen) versus "good" estrogen (16-hydroxy-estrogen), as metabolites of estradiol and estrone. There is a urine test you can take to diagnose this condition that measures the ratio of the two. If it's low, you are at risk for cancer. To restore balance in all these cases, you can take 200 mg of indole-3-carbinol (I3C) twice daily, which is derived from the brassica family of vegetables: broccoli, cauliflower, cabbage and brussels sprouts. Or take its metabolite, DIM (diindolemethane), which helps to break down estrogen in the liver. Another good nutrient for breaking down estrogen is calcium-d-glucarate (500 mg twice a day). Natural progesterone is also useful to counteract the hyperestrogen state and restore hormonal balance.

Menstrual Cramps

As many as 50% of women suffer from menstrual cramps caused by uterine contractions. Some cases are so severe that they send women to bed for a day or more. Cramps are often accompanied by bloating, dizziness and diarrhea.

Medical Treatment

- Birth control pills
- Anti-inflammatory medications (NSAIDs)

Natural Approaches

Essential fatty acids, especially GLA, can ease the contraction of smooth muscles. Herbs have been used for centuries to treat menstrual problems of all kinds, including cramps. The supplements for PMS will also help. In addition, try these:

Chasteberry: 40 drops of liquid in a glass of water every morning for four to six months.

False unicorn root tincture: 2–5 ml three times a day for up to two months.

Ginger: Place a warm tea pack over your lower abdomen.

Bromelain: 500–1,000 mg daily combined with 250 mg magnesium several times a day on an empty stomach .

Menstrual Irregularity

The complete lack of periods and spotting between periods are usually caused by an imbalance of estrogen or progesterone, although thyroid or even pituitary problems could also be contributing to the problem. Another type of menstrual irregularity is excessive bleeding, which is often caused by low progesterone levels relative to estrogen.

Medical Treatment

- Birth control pills
- A complete hormone evaluation and an essential fatty acid blood test done by a doctor

Natural Approaches

- Dietary modification to include more essential fatty acids
- Natural progesterone (up to 30 mg daily in cream)
- Chasteberry: 40 drops of concentrate in a glass of water every morning
- Addition of quality fats like flaxseed oil to your diet
- Avoidance of all hydrogenated fats

Polycystic Ovary Syndrome (PCOS)

PCOS is directly caused by a hormonal imbalance. With an excess of androgens or "male" hormones, the ovary's normal production of eggs is interrupted and small cysts are formed. Symptoms include irregular menstrual cycles or lack of periods entirely, infertility, facial hair growth, hair loss, acne and sometimes weight gain. If you have been told you have this condition, read Chapter 13 on blood sugar imbalances, especially the section on Syndrome X, because many women who have PCOS have glucose intolerance. Others may have low thyroid function, as well.

Medical Treatment

- Birth control pills
- Synthetic progestin (not the same as progesterone)
- Drugs that stop the androgenic (masculinizing) effects but don't get to the root of the problem

Natural Approaches

- Natural progesterone, to address this problem without the side effects of synthetic progestin
- Vitamin D therapy (up to 50,000 IU of ergocalciferol-type) and 1,500 mg of calcium daily, to help normalize menstrual cycles and stop excessive bleeding
- D-chiro-inositol (1,200 mg per day), to help you resume ovulation

In addition to these natural treatments, address the thyroid and insulin imbalances (see Chapters 12 and 13).

Endometriosis

Endometriosis is a painful condition that occurs when tissue from the endometrium or lining of the uterus escapes from the uterus, settling in the pelvic area or even farther away. Because the tissue is controlled by the normal hormonal fluctuations of your cycle, it grows and sometimes attaches itself to intestines, the outside of the uterus or other organs, causing pain, menstrual dysfunction, bowel pain and even infertility. The cause of endometriosis is unknown, although it is often associated with candida or yeast overgrowth (see Chapter 14). There is some evidence that estrogen dominance has a role here, as it does in so many female disorders.

Medical Treatment

- Birth control pills

- Standard hormone replacement therapy (HRT) such as Premarin

- Synthetic progesterone

- Induction of temporary menopause with such drugs as Lupron (**Caution:** this can have negative effects on breast tissue, ranging from breast tenderness to breast cancer.)

Natural Approaches

- Natural progesterone

- I3C (indole-3-carbinol) or DIM (diindolemethane): The active ingredient found in cruciferous vegetables like broccoli and cabbage that has been found to be effective for preventing breast cancer

PERIMENOPAUSE AND MENOPAUSE

Remember 51-year-old Alicia? She was sitting in my office having hot flashes and despairing over her night sweats, her cranky mood and her extra weight.

If you recognize any of Alicia's symptoms in yourself, take this little quiz:

In the past two weeks, have you experienced any of the following?

1. Broken out in profuse sweating for no apparent reason;

2. Kicked the covers off and put them on again so many times your bed looks like a helicopter has been there;

3. Been more cranky than usual with your significant other;

4. Craved chocolate (more than usual);

5. Become upset over something that wasn't really important in the big picture;

6. Lain awake at night for no apparent reason;

7. Had aching joints;

8. Had a severe headache;

9. Had heart palpitations or

10. Been uninterested in your mate's sexual advances

Total up your "yes" answers.

Got more than two?

Congratulations! You're about to join 31 million of your sisters in the adventure of a lifetime: menopause.

If you cringed and wailed, "Oh, no, not me! I'm too young for this," think again. Many women begin to experience the symptoms of perimenopause (the period when hormones begin to fluctuate before actual menopause begins) in their late thirties. More typically, symptoms of perimenopause begin after the age of 40.

Perimenopause, which can last anywhere from one to ten years or more, marks the beginning of the time when your hormone production begins to fall or become unpredictable. Our moms used to call it "the change." You could hear the dread in their voices. To them, menopause meant going slightly nuts. It meant periods from hell, then no periods at all. It led to changing sweat-soaked bed sheets twice a night, tirades aimed at uncomprehending family members and floods of tears, not to speak of those menopausal five pounds a year. It may even have meant becoming old before their time.

Now that it's upon you, take heart. Remember, this is *not* your mother's menopause. Fortunately, you live in the 21st century, and we have solutions.

In fact, menopause isn't a disease. It's a rite of passage. It happens to every woman, and a vast majority of women report being the happiest and most fulfilled of any period of their lives between the ages of 50 and 65. Usually (we hope!) it coincides with the departure of children from the household and a new era in your life when your time becomes your own again.

We shouldn't treat it as an illness, either. Ancient spiritual practices revere the crone as the woman who has lived long enough to truly know herself; the woman who enjoys sex for its pure pleasure without fear of pregnancy; the woman whose wisdom is sought by her family, friends and community.

What's Happening in Your Body?

Technically, perimenopause means you are beginning to ovulate irregularly. Your ovaries have released just about all of the viable eggs you were born with. That means a slowing down of your body's natural production of two essential hormones: estrogen and progesterone. You start to have cycles where no egg is released, called anovulatory cycles. As a result, there is not progesterone to smooth out the estrogen, and you are in an estrogen-dominant state. Or your estrogen may become so low that your pituitary gland starts sending out signals to your ovaries, via the hormone FSH, to produce more estrogen. Sometimes your ovaries go along with the message, but sometimes they don't, so your hormones fluctuate by the month, by the day, and even by the hour.

The list goes on and on. Each woman has her own perimenopause. Some of us experience barely noticeable symptoms, and some of us get the screaming meemies. Most of us fall somewhere in the middle with one or two symptoms becoming particularly bothersome as we move from perimenopause to menopause (medically defined as the absence of menstrual periods for 12 months).

If you've already gone 12 months without a period, naturally or through surgical intervention, you're fully menopausal.

Measuring Hormone Levels

There are laboratory tests, including some good home tests, to help you get a general picture of your hormone levels. Discuss the need for a complete hormone profile with your doctor. Many doctors prefer to test only estrogen levels, but these don't give a full picture of your hormonal status. For my perimenopausal patients I will check blood levels of estrogen, progesterone, DHEA-S, testosterone, pregnenolone, FSH, LH, and SHBG. These tests can be fairly expensive, but the results are worth it. Another route is saliva, for which you can order a home test kit, and yet another, 24 hour urine test, which is the most comprehensive, and requires a doctor's prescription.

If you haven't already taken one of these tests, consider it now.

If you have mild symptoms, for example, a few simple hot flashes and you're pretty sure what's causing them, go ahead to the treatment section and see if one or more of the options there gives you relief. If you still need fine-tuning, you might need to take one of these tests later.

In any case, treatment for perimenopausal symptoms and menopause are pretty much the same, with the exception that as perimenopause progresses, your dosages may change. You can take saliva, urine or blood tests to determine the levels of hormones in your system. There is some controversy about the relative accuracy of these tests, with some experts considering a saliva test to be more accurate because it measures the "unbound" or "free" hormones. This is the amount actually available for action on the cells, an important factor when you want to determine precise dosages for purposes of hormone replacement.

Blood tests, on the other hand, will measure total estrogen, both bound and unbound or free. Blood tests may be more accurate, particularly in a woman who has already begun taking hormone replacement therapy. For the sake of convenience, though, the less expensive saliva test can be used as a baseline. Follow-up testing can be with blood tests, which are more expensive and require a prescription. Saliva tests may still be useful at that point. Or get a 24 hour urine test, generally prescribed by doctors who are more holistically oriented; e.g. Meridian Valley Labs (www.meridianvalleylab.com) or Genova Diagnostics (www. gdx.com)

By measuring the blood level of sex hormone binding globulin (SHBG), you can determine the blood serum's capacity to keep the hormone bound and unavailable for use.

At the very least, if you think you have hormone-related problems, the following are the basic ones to check.

Because your hormones will fluctuate over the course of the month, take blood or urine tests on days 19–21 of your cycle, called the "luteal phase," with day 1 being the first day of your period. If you are cycling, regular or not, take a series of samples that covers a month's time and will show fluctuations. If you're irregular, do your best estimate for urine or blood tests, or a one-shot saliva test. If you're still cycling, the estrogen and progesterone are best taken at intervals throughout the month in order to track your monthly pattern. The kit supplies extra tubes and instructions for this. If you are menopausal, it doesn't matter when you take the tests.

Here are the plasma ranges for these tests. Saliva and urine tests will have different ranges. Remember that your hormone levels fluctuate daily and even throughout the day. These values show broad ranges, and what's normal for someone else may not be for you.

Estradiol: normal range is 150–750 pg/mL for nonmenopausal women at midcycle (day 14) and less than 20 pg/mL for menopausal women. We may test for the other forms of estrogen if necessary, but usually just estradiol will do.

Progesterone: normal range is .2–28 ng/mL for nonmenopausal women, depending on the time in the cycle (3.3–25.6 is considered normal for the luteal phase or peak), and 0–.7 for postmenopausal women. This drops in the time between ovulation and the first day of your period to less than 10 ng/mL.

Total testosterone: normal range is 14–76 ng/dL for premenopausal women and 5–51 for menopausal women.

You'll get additional information if you add these tests, which do not shift during the menstrual cycle:

DHEA-S (an adrenal hormone that may also convert to male or female hormones in the cells, depending your own body's chemistry): normal range for women ages 19 to 30 is 29–781 mcg/dL and for women 31 to 50 is 12–379. Postmenopausal normal range is 30–260.

Cortisol (the stress hormone): in a blood test taken in the morning, normal range is 4.3–22.4 mcg/dL, and for an evening test, the normal range is 3.1–16.7. Saliva tests may take four readings over the course of the day to observe your pattern.

Medical Management

Equine-Based Hormone Replacement (Premarin, Prempro)

The HRT decision is a difficult one, made even more difficult by the disturbing results of the Women's Health Initiative, a large scientific study sponsored by the National Institutes of Health. The study was stopped in July 2002 after preliminary results showed that the group of women taking taking Prempro, a pharmaceutical HRT (a horse urine-based estrogen, plus a synthetic hormone called progestin that supposedly mimics progesterone) offered no protection against disease, as doctors had long believed. Results showed that the women taking the combination actually had 27% *more* heart attacks than those who got the placebo. They also had a higher rate of breast cancer, which wasn't really a surprise. That's not to speak of 38% more strokes and more than double the number of blood clots. A later study suggested pharmaceutical HRT may also double the risk of Alzheimer's disease in women over 65.

Unfortunately, many women and most of the medical establishment think the only way to treat the symptoms of menopause is with formulas made from the urine of pregnant horses. And they want to protect against uterine cancer with a synthetic version of progesterone called progestin.

Women aren't horses and our hormonal makeup is vastly different. While horse urine may be effective at easing some of the more unpleasant symptoms of menopause, the science is now solid: pharmaceutical HRT increases your risk of serious disease. In three words: *Don't take it!*

Horse urine contains estrone, one of the major estrogens found in humans, and it contains equilin, another type of estrogen not found in humans. These drugs have little resemblance to the hormonal makeup of a human female. It's no wonder that these compounds have played havoc with women's health for 60 years!

Plus, progestin and progesterone are as different as day and night. Progestin has been linked to a large number of side effects, including increased depression and mood swings, water retention, heart disease, strokes and even uterine cancer. Natural progesterone, on the other hand, actually protects you against uterine cancer. It also helps build strong bones and even helps our bodies create other hormones when we need them.

There are natural forms of complete hormone replacement that don't have the risks of the pharmaceuticals.

Natural Ways to Balance Sex Hormones

First remember that, just as with every other health condition we're addressing in this book, every woman's menopause or perimenopause needs to be treated in an individual manner. There is no such thing as a one-size-fits-all hormone solution.

One of the simplest ways to deal with perimenopause is through your food intake: Lots and lots and lots of fresh fruits and vegetables will go a long way toward eliminating the annoying symptoms of menopause and keeping your sex hormones balanced.

That may work for you, or you may need to also consider other possibilities.

For example, now that we've said all those bad things about synthetic hormone replacement, let us put in a plug for hormone replacement of the right kind.

If you're starting to think estrogen, progesterone and other hormones are all "bad," consider this: Extensive research proves estrogen protects us from heart disease, osteoporosis, colon cancer and Alzheimer's disease. What's more, estrogen is proved to have a positive effect on mental clarity, sexuality and libido, skin health, emotional health and digestion.

In addition, studies prove that progesterone helps prevent uterine cancer and possibly breast cancer, supports proper thyroid and blood sugar function and helps create other hormones as needed.

You *can* have it all through *bio-identical hormones,* compounds that naturally duplicate hormones exactly as your body manufactured them at its prime. The term *bio-identical* was coined by naturopathic physician Marcus Laux, author of *Natural Woman, Natural Menopause* (1998).

Bio-identical hormones are derived from soy and wild yams by a complex manufacturing process that transforms them into a carbon copy of the hormones you had at your peak of hormone production. They're not plant or herbal extracts, but are called *natural* both because of their natural origin and their molecular structure.

Your body has a lock-and-key mechanism for hormonal activity. To put it simply, your body either manufactures hormones or you take them as supplements. They are supposed to fit perfectly into receptors, like keys. Bio-identical hormones fit exactly into those receptors, while synthetic ones don't fit exactly. Others can stay too long or not long enough, making your symptoms and your long-term risks worse. For details on these hormones and how they are prescribed, see Dr. Uzzi Reiss's excellent books, *Natural Hormone Balance for Women* (Atria, 2002) and his latest, *The Natural Superwoman* (Avery, 2008).

Your doctor probably won't mention this to you because most likely, he or she doesn't know about these natural hormones that have been available for about 20 years. But do ask about them, because you can get natural hormones only by prescription. Just like any other prescription drug, their manufacture is regulated for safety and efficacy by the FDA.

If your doctor is not familiar with natural hormone replacement, you may meet with resistance. Even in the wake of the Women's Health Initiative, many doctors will still insist that equine estrogens and progestin are the standard. The fact is, they are neither the standard nor good enough for you! There are compounding pharmacies that can supply them to order, based on your individual hormonal needs. There are many excellent compounding pharmacies, with more opening all the time. A list of pharmacies is available in Chapter 18 or check with the International Academy of Compounding Pharmacists. Contact: (IACP) at www.iacprx.org.

Most will do mail order, so there is no need for them to be nearby. They can be excellent resources for information. Some, such as Women's International Pharmacy, have lists of doctors all over the country who prescribe natural hormone replacement. Call (800) 279-5708, or go to www.womensinternational. com.

Bio-identical hormones are by no means the only natural way of addressing perimenopause and menopause. Consider the following well-tested herbs and supplements:

Black Cohosh (*cimecifuga racemosa*): This is the gold standard for treating many symptoms of perimenopause and menopause, and we recommend you try this one first. It's extremely effective against hot flashes. Black cohosh is also useful to combat fatigue, irritability, mood swings, night sweats, headaches and insomnia. One of the most widely studied herbs to address these symptoms, it is also helpful in stabilizing blood pressure and relieving heart palpitations.
Cautions: Rarely, stomach discomfort,
Dosage: Take 20–100 mg twice daily of extract standardized to 1 mg 26-deoxyacteine per 20 mg tablet or capsule

Soy isoflavones: Soy is a rich source of plant estrogens that have a structure similar to human estrogen and affect the way estrogen is metabolized in your body without negative side effects. Recent British research shows that the isoflavones in soy may help prevent breast cancer while reducing the risk of heart disease and osteoporosis.

Cautions: More is not better. Excessive soy has its downside: Too much estrogen relative to other hormones can be as problematic as not having enough. If you are on kidney dialysis or if you have had a hormonally-related cancer or are risk for one (breast, ovarian), talk to your doctor before taking soy isoflavones.

Dosage: 100 mg per day.

Chasteberry (*vitex agnus castus*): This herb has been used for centuries to help banish those vicious mood swings during perimenopause by balancing your estrogen and progesterone levels. It can also help relieve hot flashes. Vitex also helps support normal menstrual functions, so it can help relieve heavy and irregular periods, enhance skin health and balance the function of the pituitary gland.

Cautions: Chasteberry has, on rare occasions, been known to cause headaches, weight gain, nausea and diarrhea. The side effects disappear quickly once you stop taking it. Do not take chasteberry if you are pregnant, might become pregnant or are taking hormone therapies of any kind, including thyroid medications or antidepressants.

Dosage: 20–120 mg per day in capsule form or as a liquid extract according to manufacturer's instructions.

Red clover (*trifolium pratense*): This is a rich source of isoflavones, the same compounds found in soy, which stimulate the ovaries to increase estrogen production, maximizing what you have, even in perimenopause. Red clover's isoflavones will help protect you against heart disease and osteoporosis.

Cautions: None.

Dosage: 1 to 3 grams daily.

Licorice (*glycyrrhiza glabria*): The tasty herb lowers estradiol levels while raising progesterone levels, helping reduce a broad range of menopausal symptoms, especially hot flashes and fatigue, since it helps boost energy levels by stimulating the adrenal gland. It has also been used traditionally to combat depression.

Cautions: Women at risk for estrogen sensitive cancers should not use licorice, nor should people with high blood pressure, kidney problems or abnormally low potassium levels.

Dosage: Use glycyrrhizin extract, 200–1,000 mg of glycyrrhizin extract (the active ingredient in licorice) daily, depending on severity of symptoms for up to 6 weeks. Resume, if necessary, after a two-week break.

CoenzymeQ$_{10}$: CoQ$_{10}$ is your body's energy catalyst—the beginning point of a chain of chemical reactions that creates the energy your cells needs to function at optimal level. It's also a powerful antioxidant that gobbles up disease-causing free radicals. It's particularly important in preventing heart disease and treating existing heart disease.
Cautions: Can cause mild gastrointestinal upset.
Dosage: 60–100 mg twice daily. CoQ$_{10}$ is fat-soluble and should be taken as a softgel for best absorption and utilization.

Carnitine: L-carnitine as it's officially named addresses a host of peri-menopausal and menopausal complaints. It's found in natural meat and dairy products, less so in the hormone- and antibiotic-laden products you find in the supermarket today. You probably need it even if you're not a vegetarian. It is widely used to improve brain function and mental sharpness, assist in weight loss and increase general energy levels. Because carnitine helps all cells to use their energy more efficiently, it also helps your body stay young. If that's not enough, it also helps keep blood fats (triglycerides) low and HDL or "good" cholesterol high, just where you want them.
Cautions: At higher dosages, carnitine can cause gastrointestinal problems. If this happens, lower the dosage and gradually build back up to your optimal level. Avoid taking it after 3 p.m. because it may be too stimulating and interfere with sleep. Some people report vivid dreaming, so adjust your dose accordingly.
Dosage: From 500 to 4,000 mg daily, depending on your purpose in using the supplement. Go toward the higher end for weight loss or if your doctor has told you that you have seriously high triglycerides.

Dong quai (*angelica sinensis*): This fragrant herb has been used in Asia for centuries to relieve hot flashes, mood swings, insomnia, night sweats and headaches.
Cautions: Because dong quai enhances estrogen production, it can intensify

bleeding, so do not use this herb during your menstrual period if you have heavy bleeding.

Dosage: 200 mg three times a day.

DHEA: If your lab tests have shown your DHEA levels are low, DHEA supplements may help bring you back into balance and help relieve stress. Your body also converts DHEA into estrogen, progesterone and testosterone, and each of us will have more of one pathway than another. Some of my patients turn it into estrogen, while others, testosterone.

Cautions: DHEA levels should be monitored by your doctor since it does convert to other hormones and may cause unwanted side effects. There is a possibility that in the presence of cancer, it may enhance abnormal cell growth.

Dosage: Usually you'll need between 5 to 25 mg daily, but that is dependent on your lab results, and you should take it under the supervision of your doctor.

Address That Menopausal Weight Gain

We wish we could tell you there's an easy solution to the problem of menopausal weight gain, but there isn't. Our metabolism slows as we age, and a certain amount of weight gain is hard to avoid. (See Chapter 17 for general guidelines on weight management as well as a list of supplements to take.)

Some experts suggest that our satiety or "fullness" indicators may become dulled over time, and even more so as our hormone levels begin to fall. In simple terms, this means we often eat when we are already full. It may help to put your food on the plate and stop when it's gone, even if you think you still want more.

The mini-meal plan in which you eat several small meals throughout the day is a good bet for those of us who have gained weight as our hormones have tapered off. A steady intake of calories also keeps blood sugars stable and prevents cravings and energy swings, and the constant intake of small amounts of food balances all our hormones.

These supplements can help:

Carnitine: See the section above. Some experts say a deficiency of this amino acid contained in meat is a major cause of weight gain. Carnitine is responsible for revving up the fat burning furnaces. It's also great for your heart, brain function, builds energy and reduces stress.

Cautions: Can cause gastrointestinal problems at high dosages. Build up your dosage gradually. Some people report exceptionally vivid dreams, which might be a good thing!

Dosage: You'll need at least 1,000 mg of L-carnitine daily. You can safely take up to 4,000 mg

Carb blockers: Phase 2 (short for Phaseolamin 2250™, which is how you'll see it listed on bottles sold under a number of brand names), this supplement derived from white kidney beans can safely block your body's absorption of starchy carbohydrates by 66%. Italian studies show that Phase 2 neutralizes as many as 2,250 carb calories in a day, so they pass right through your system without being converted to sugar and becoming fat. It doesn't work with pure sugars, as in cookies and cake, just starches.

Cautions: May cause mild gas and bloating.

Dosage: Take between 1,000 and 1,500 mg before each of your two meals highest in carbohydrates.

Glutamine: This amino acid curbs sugar and salt cravings by as much as 50%! In addition, glutamine naturally elevates levels of growth hormone in your body, making your cells multiply faster. Additional amounts of growth hormone help mobilize fat from storage, like on your hips and thighs and makes it available for energy.

Cautions: Do not use if you have kidney or liver disease.

Dosage: 200 mg to 1 gram with water 30 minutes before meals.

Essential Fatty Acids: Fats release the hormone cholecystokinin from the stomach to the brain, telling you that you are full and keeping you feeling full for up to six hours after you eat.

Cautions: None.

Dosage: Look for a combination essential fatty acids that contains Omega- 3 and 6 Take at least 1,000 mg capsule or 1 tablespoon of liquid twice daily. Keep refrigerated to prevent rancidity.

Chromium: Chromium is a vital mineral that helps turn carbohydrates into glucose, the fuel burned by your cells for energy. It helps regulate insulin, a hormone that helps control hunger, fat storage and muscle building. Chromium also increases the power of insulin to produce the brain chemical serotonin, which numerous studies have proven curbs appetite, as well as improves mood.
Cautions: Rarely: Sleep irregularities, palpitations .
Dosage: Take up to 200–500 mcg a day of chromium picolinate or niconate for eight weeks. Chromium picolinate includes picolinic acid, another stimulator of brain chemicals that soothe nerves and curb appetite. Chromium nicotinate contains niacin, known to lower cholesterol.

Natural Ways to Restore Sex Drive

These time-tested and scientifically validated remedies can help restore your sex drive:

Tango: This old Chinese remedy recently became available in the U.S, and it's a great way to increase sexual desire and pleasure. It also helps you reach orgasm and helps you reach stronger and longer orgasms. A mélange of chrysanthemum flowers, cinnamon, three types of mushrooms, ginseng, licorice and more, Tango is a very effective way of getting things going, quickly. Take a capsule or two and in a couple of hours, you and your partner should be ready to go. (You can get it at www.drcass.com)
Cautions: Do not use if you are pregnant or nursing.
Dosage: One capsule as needed, or for long-term effects, take a capsule every day.

Damiana (*Turnera diffusa, aphrodisiaca*): Also useful for headaches, some studies suggest that this South American may work like testosterone in enhancing libido. It is best known as an aphrodisiac, so fasten your seat belt, it's time to enjoy sex again! It is also a useful antidepressant, and it can help break the cycle of depression = low sexual desire = depression.
Cautions: None known, but if it doesn't relieve your symptoms in six weeks, try something else.
Dosage: 3–4 grams daily.

Maca root and deer antler: Great libido boosters! Both stimulate hormone production and enhance stamina for great sex.
Cautions: None at recommended dosages.
Dosage: Take 300 mg of maca daily and increase dosage to three times a day, if necessary. Take up to 1,000 mg of deer antler daily. They work well in combination.

Muira puama: Improves circulation to the pelvis and genitals and works well with maca or deer antler because their effects enhance one another.
Cautions: None
Dosage: 1–3 ml of a 4:1 tincture twice daily.

Natural testosterone: This hormone improves your sex drive and sexual pleasure two- to three-fold. You can get natural testosterone with a prescription at compounding pharmacies, preferably as a topical cream, applied to the smooth skin areas of the body, as thinly spread as possible for maximum absorption. You can use it as a lubricant if vaginal dryness is a problem. It works better when combined with estrogen. Remember, hormones should be tested and prescribed accordingly.
Cautions: None at the recommended dosage. Excesssive amounts can cause acne, excessive facial hair growth, and aggressive behavior.
Dosage: Start with a low concentration of 1–2 mg per gram of cream and use it every other day. You may need more or less, but can monitor both your response and at intervals, lab tests.

These remedies aren't anything like taking an aspirin and expecting your headache will disappear in a few minutes. If you decide to try any of them, give them 2–6 weeks to work. Many natural remedies, particularly herbs, take longer to work than pharmaceuticals because they are bringing about fundamental changes in your body, so be patient.
Also consider these:

- Yoga, meditation, massage: anything that chills you out and pampers you will ease the stressfulness of these difficult times, so indulge!

- Exercise of any type will help your body regain its natural balance.

12

THYROID AND ADRENALS: YOUR ENERGY GLANDS

If your journey to find a cause of your exhaustion and a dozen other puzzling symptoms has led you to this section, welcome. You may be about to find some connections among the mishmash of strange and seemingly unrelated symptoms that probably have plagued you for years.

More than 10 million adult Americans have thyroid disease. Another 13 million are estimated to have undiagnosed thyroid insufficiencies. A significant number of women have "subclinical" or "below the radar" hypothyroidism, in which blood tests may be normal or have only slightly elevated levels of a hormone called thyroid-stimulating hormone (TSH). The only symptom may be fatigue. Of people with this condition, 2% progress to full-blown hypothyroidism each year. The numbers are much more sobering for older women, with 17% of subclinical cases developing hypothyroidism each year.

Adrenal imbalance is on the rise because of the levels of chronic and even toxic stress we experience in modern society.

We've put these two conditions together because the symptoms, and the treatments, can be quite similar. Every process that goes on inside our bodies requires energy and specifically, metabolic energy. When your body doesn't have enough energy to function properly, you're like a car with a sputtering engine. It just can't get up and go like it should!

HYPOTHYROIDISM
(LOW THYROID FUNCTION)

Here is the sequence of events that tells us how the thyroid controls energy production in the cells. The thyroid gland, located at the base of the neck, makes the hormone T4 (thyroxine). T4 is converted in the thyroid and the liver to its active form, T3 (triiodothyronine), which then turns on the energy production inside every cell of the body. The output of thyroid hormones is controlled by TSH (thyroid-stimulating hormone), which is released by the pituitary gland, located in the brain, behind the forehead. The pituitary takes its orders from a part of the brain called the hypothalamus.

The tiny adrenal glands, located on top of each kidney, help the body deal with stress. If the metabolic activity is too high, the adrenals perceive this as a stress and send a message to the hypothalamus, which then will cause the pituitary to produce less TSH, which slows down the thyroid.

If your energy has slowed down it can be due to any of the following:

- The thyroid gland can't make enough T4.

- The T4 is not being converted to its active form, T3.

- The adrenal glands become too weak to handle the body's normal rate of metabolism so they go on strike and force a slowdown in energy production.

- The enzymes (cellular machinery) that make ATP may be held back due to chemical interference such as toxins, lack of needed nutrients or breakdown due to autoimmune disease or viral damage.

- Imbalances in hormones such as estrogen, progesterone or testosterone can affect energy production.

- Starvation leads to energy slowdown, which explains why it's not good to fast for prolonged periods.

The bottom line: every cell of your body needs thyroid hormone to function properly, and so when thyroid function is impaired, nothing in your whole body is running at its optimal level. We seem to be seeing more hypothyroidism, which many experts think is a result of our fast-paced lifestyle.

Tired and Cold

Lisa's story is quite typical. A 35-year-old legal assistant and mother of two, she told me that it took a while for the red flags to pop up. First it was a little weight gain. Then it was a feeling of fatigue, which she credited to "getting older." She had trouble getting out of bed in the morning despite sleeping eight hours, and she needed to jump-start herself with a strong cup of coffee.

I stopped her with an odd question: "Do you wear socks to bed?"

"How did you know?" she asked.

"Because you have many of the other symptoms of thyroid imbalance," I answered, "and this one is almost a sure sign of low thyroid function. The other clue is the 'gotta have' your morning coffee." It turned out that her mother had also had hypothyroidism, ever since the birth of her third child. In fact, Lisa's problem began after her last pregnancy—a common starting point for many women.

Lisa's symptoms were fairly typical. Thyroid imbalances can manifest in dozens of different ways, from a few symptoms to a dozen or more.

Here's a partial list of the most common symptoms of thyroid imbalance:

- Gain in weight that is difficult to lose
- Fatigue, especially in the morning
- Trouble getting up in the morning
- Excessive sleeping
- Digestive problems and constipation
- Feeling cold, especially hands and feet
- Moodiness and depression
- Brain fog: poor memory and concentration
- Low sex drive
- Low body temperature
- Brittle nails
- Dry skin
- Thinning and/or coarse hair

- Thinning of outer edge of eyebrows
- Headaches
- Low, husky voice
- Muscle and joint aches and pains
- Menstrual changes or fertility problems
- Lowered resistance to/increased numbers of infections
- Tinnitus (ringing in the ears)
- Allergies
- Heart palpitations
- Slow pulse and low blood pressure
- High cholesterol and triglycerides
- Sleep apnea and snoring
- Shortness of breath
- Tightness in the chest
- Dizziness and vertigo
- Carpal tunnel syndrome
- Puffiness and swelling of face, feet or hands

Having even two or three of these symptoms is an indication that your thyroid is likely not functioning properly.

Causes of Hypothyroidism

Hypothyroidism can be caused by any number of factors, starting with genetics. I always ask patients whom I suspect of having hypothyroidism if there is a family history, and very often the answer is yes, with mothers, grandmothers, and sisters having had it. Be extra vigilant if it runs in your family.

Other causes include surgical removal of the thyroid for cancer, radioactive iodine treatment for hyperthyroidism or Graves' disease, and radiation treatment to the head, neck or chest. Hypothyroidism is also often associated with autoimmune diseases or endocrine problems such as chronic fatigue and immune dysfunction syndrome (CFIDS), fibromyalgia and insulin-dependent diabetes. Other causes are chronic stress and smoking.

Certain medications, such as lithium, amiodarone (a heart drug), estrogen and sulfa drugs, can cause hypothyroidism.

The Iodine Connection

All hormone receptors need iodine before their hormones can be used. One way to boost your hormone levels is to be sure you have enough iodine. Most people don't. Despite the introduction of iodized salt, dietary shortage of iodine is still a cause of hypothyroidism. There is evidence that 12% of the U.S. population is deficient in iodine. Also, we are exposed to excessive amounts of fluoride and chloride (from tap water), bromide added to bread dough, and radioactive fallout (Yes, there is radioactive iodine in the atmosphere that we breathe, due to nuclear testing and other nuclear wastes). All of these interfere with iodine function.

Dr. Guy Abraham has done research that shows how both your thyroid and your breast tissues need iodine and iodide for normal function, and many women are deficient. Dr. Abraham has developed a 24-hour urine iodine-loading test that is available through doctors' offices, including mine, and if deficient, you need to take an iodine supplement. One that I prescribe is a combination of iodine and iodide.

Hashimoto's Autoimmune Thyroiditis

A variation of hypothyroidism is an autoimmune disorder called Hashimoto's autoimmune thyroiditis. In addition to the usual symptoms, those with this disorder may experience mood swings and bursts of energy or anxiety for no reason, as well as insomnia, heartbeat irregularities, and even panic attacks. I have seen women with this disorder misdiagnosed as having bipolar disorder. Hashimoto's thyroiditis is diagnosed by the presence of antibodies—antimicrosomal and antithyroglobulin—to the thyroid hormones. The treatment is the same as for hypothyroidism, with the addition of anti-inflammatory supplements. The response to the treatment must be monitored carefully to keep a balance between under- and overactivity.

Here is a situation that I see all too often: Joanne consulted me after a clean bill of health from her endocrinologist. She described herself as feeling depressed, irritable, "like I'm jumping out of my skin," and at the same time, exhausted. She had read something I'd written on the subject, and came to me as her last resort. She brought in the lab results from the endocrinologist. Her TSH was 4.8, not high enough for him to want to give her a hypothyroid diagnosis, though I would have, and her T3 and T4 were in normal range. When I tested her antibody levels, which had not been done, they were quite high. Joanne did indeed suffer from Hashimoto's thyroiditis, which responded well to treatment: 1 grain of natural dessicated thyroid daily, which contains both T3 and T4, 3 g of fish oil daily for the inflammation, a multivitamin, and a variety of antioxidants.

Testing and Diagnosis

Diagnosing hypothyroidism is difficult because standard tests don't always provide the information you're seeking. There are also the relative values of each of the hormones, T3, T4, and TSH, which tell a more complete story. For an excellent description and chart, see www.drrind.com.

Basal Body Temperature

This simple test using an ordinary oral mercury thermometer will let you know if your thyroid may be sluggish and require further investigation.

Shake the thermometer down the night before because you should be in a resting mode for the test. When you first awaken, before you get out of bed, place the mercury thermometer in your armpit. A digital thermometer won't give an accurate underarm reading. Leave it there for 10 minutes, and then record your reading. Take the reading at the same time every day for the next four days. If you are still in your menstrual years, begin on the third day of your period. Don't take it close to or during ovulation when your temperature is highest. If you are no longer menstruating, you can take it at any time of the month.

If your reading is consistently below 97.8 degrees, it's possible you have hypothyroidism. Repeat the test for at least three mornings (close in time, if not consecutive), and take an average. If you are on a thyroid treatment program, take your temperatures monthly to monitor your progress.

Thyroid Blood Tests

Testing blood levels of TSH (the hormone that is stimulating your thyroid to produce more thyroid hormone) and T4 (the major thyroid hormone) may be helpful. A high level of TSH indicates your thyroid function is too low. A normal TSH range is considered to be between .35 and 5.5. Optimal level is under 2. If you are above 2, you may have an underactive thyroid gland, although the majority of doctors feel that you need a higher TSH to qualify. There are homes tests available.

I have seen countless women patients over the years whose doctors told them their tests were normal or borderline low and refused to treat them, even though they had clear symptoms of hypothyroidism. Most thyroid tests today are not sensitive enough to identify borderline cases or mild thyroid malfunction. You may be very low in thyroid hormone and still have normal lab tests. Also, individuals can differ in what is a "normal" reading for them.

Because you are now fairly sure your problem is a thyroid imbalance, take these additional tests. Although many conventional doctors will balk at this, I have seen many patients who show normal TSH levels and abnormal results in the following tests:

- **T4 or total thyroxine:** normal range is approximately 4.5–12.0. A reading of less than 4.5, along with high TSH, may indicate hypothyroidism. A low T4 with low TSH may indicate a pituitary problem.

- **Free T4:** normal range is 0.7–1.53. Less than 0.7 may indicate hypothyroidism.

- **Total T3:** normal range is approximately 60–181 ng/dL. Less than 60 may indicate hypothyroidism. Optimal is 120–124.

- **Free T3:** normal range is approximately 260–480 pg/mL. Less than 260 may indicate hypothyroidism.

- **Reverse T3:** this is a "false" T3 that the body produces during times of chronic stress or starvation (or "overdieting"). It takes up space on theT3 receptors, blocking the real T3 and preventing energy production. It's like applying the brakes in order to decrease energy expenditure.

- **Antithyroid antibodies:** antibodies to thyroperoxidase (TPO) or thyroglobulin (TG) will be elevated in Hashimoto's autoimmune thyroiditis.

While these tests may be helpful, they may not give you the results you are seeking. TSH and T4, in particular, can appear normal even when a severe deficiency exists.

Low morning body temperature is a major indicator of hypothyroidism, and that in itself may be sufficient reason to begin taking thyroid medication. Continue to check your basal body temperature throughout your Vibrant Health Plan to monitor the success of the things you're doing to address your imbalance.

In the end, find a doctor who's willing to give you a low dosage of thyroid hormone based on your symptoms, and see if you get relief. Untreated thyroid disease can lead to anemia, low body temperature, depression, and, in the extreme, heart failure.

An excellent website about thyroid and adrenal function, including information on how to interpret your test results, is www.drrine.com.

Conventional Medical Treatment

Medications most commonly prescribed for hypothyroidism are Synthroid, Levoxyl, or Unithroid, brand names for the generic levothyroxine. They contain synthetic T4. Most doctors prefer to begin a newly diagnosed patient with a low dose and gradually increase the dosage until TSH levels return to normal. It's important to carefully monitor the dosage because excessive amounts of thyroid hormones can lead to symptoms of hyperthyroidism.

Synthroid is taken by eight million Americans and, thanks to an extensive advertising campaign, is the third-bestselling medication in the United States. It is no more effective than the two other major brands, although it is more expensive.

Because levothyroxine is simply T4, it works well only for those whose bodies can effectively convert the T4 to T3. Often, patients taking synthetic hormones need additional T3. That is available as Cytomel or as time-released, compounded liothyronine, which I use in my practice and comes from a compounding pharmacy. There is also a synthetic T4/T3 drug called Thyrolar, which can be substituted for the two once the correct doses of each have been established.

If you take a higher dose than you need, these medications can cause symptoms of hyperthyroidism: heart palpitations, angina, atrial fibrillation, heart failure, heat intolerance, headache, insomnia, menstrual irregularity, nausea, vomiting, diarrhea and hair loss. In addition, they can reduce the effectiveness of several medications, including estrogens, anticoagulants and beta-blockers. Caution: Don't take thyroid hormone at the same time as calcium or iron because they interfere with its absorption. Leave about half an hour between them.

Natural Thyroid Hormones

Natural thyroid hormones are available by prescription under the brand names Armour Thyroid, Westhroid and Naturethroid. Made from the desiccated thyroid glands of pigs (sorry, but pigs do have a similar physiology to humans), they all contain the complete range of thyroid hormone components including T4 and T3. Naturethroid is hypoallergenic and doesn't contain derivatives of corn, a common allergen. It's what I prescribe in my practice.

I prefer these "old-time" remedies, in use for more than a hundred years, because my patients do so well on them. I have also seen my patients do poorly when they switched to synthetic thyroid hormones. Many doctors are reluctant to prescribe these natural thyroid preparations because they have been told they are impure and the dosage is not consistent. I have not found that to be true. More information is available to you and your doctor on the Broda Barnes Foundation website: www.brodabarnes.org.

If the T3 is still low, I will add a small dose of time-released T3 from a compounding pharmacy. I prefer this to Cytomel, which is released more quickly and can sometimes cause a period of agitation soon after taking it, followed by a drop in energy as it wears off. T3 enhances serotonin content in the brain, elevating mood and enhancing sleep. In fact, the SSRI antidepressants such Prozac, Zoloft and Lexapro may produce some of their effects by raising the availability of T3 in the brain.

There are no over-the-counter thyroid medications. There are some over-the-counter and multilevel marketing "glandular" supplements that have varying amounts of thyroid hormone.

Optimal intake of vitamins A, C, and E, vitamin B complex, especially B_{12}, plus magnesium, manganese, selenium, zinc, and coenzyme Q_{10} is important for thyroid balance. Dosages should match those in recommended multivitamins.

Here are some natural supplements that can help balance thyroid function. In all these treatments, look out for signs of overstepping the balance point, into thyroid hyperactivity. Symptoms include insomnia, irritability, weight loss, heat sensitivity, increased perspiration, muscular weakness, visual changes, lighter menstrual flow, rapid heartbeat and hand tremors.

Iodine: Thyroid problems can be caused by a deficiency of iodine. Scientific evidence shows that 12% of the U.S., population is deficient in iodine, despite its presence in most table salt. Iodine and herbal remedies like kelp, bladderwrack and bugleweed may help some people with hypothyroidism and make matters worse for others. You'll need to self-monitor on this one.
Cautions: None at the recommended dosage.
Dosage: 1 mg per day.

Tyrosine: This amino acid is one of the building blocks of thyroid hormone as well as the brain chemicals dopamine, norepinephrine and epinephrine. It is known to have a positive effect on thyroid function.
Cautions: Mild gastrointestinal discomfort in some people. Check with your doctor if you have high blood pressure.
Dosage: 500–1,000 mg twice daily.

Dietary Solutions

In addition to your healthy diet, avoid excessive intake of raw broccoli, cabbage, cauliflower, mustard, millet, and other foods known as goitrogenics (literally, "causing goiter", or hypothyroidism). You are in no danger at a serving or two a day, and cooked foods in this category are fine because cooking inactivates the compounds that may cause thyroid imbalance.

Soy-based foods present a dilemma because some experts believe soy increases metabolic rate and thyroid function, and others indicate high soy intake, especially in supplement form, may make matters worse. The biggest danger here is to infants fed with soy-based formula, because it has been shown to lead to thyroid problems in later life, such as autoimmune thyroiditis.

Some people with autoimmune thyroiditis have been found to have celiac disease, an intolerance to gluten (found in wheat, rye, barley), so do check this out.

Other Therapies That May Help

Yoga can be enormously effective in normalizing thyroid function. Particularly helpful are postures like *sarvangasana,* the shoulder stand, that send energy to the area of the thyroid. You're likely to see results if you can gradually build up your practice of this posture to 5 to 10 minutes a day,.

Back to Lisa: she had already had a TSH test, but her doctor resisted ordering the T3 and T4 tests because her TSH, at 3.7, was in the normal range. He told her to lose weight and her energy would pick up. Instead, Lisa came to me. After a short time on natural dessicated thyroid, her energy picked up, and her weight started to come off. She's much happier today! This was combined with a program that included substantial adrenal support as well, and you will see why.

ADRENALS: THE STRESS MACHINES

Before treating low thyroid, I always assess adrenal function. It's most likely low, too. By then supporting the adrenals, you can give a good boost to the thyroid. Conversely, if you treat only the thyroid but not the adrenals, you can end up overstimulating the already overworked adrenals, creating even more imbalance in your system.

The tiny adrenal glands perched atop the kidneys produce a number of important hormones. The core or medulla makes adrenaline (epinephrine), the fight-or-flight stress hormone.

The outer part of the adrenal gland, the cortex, makes the following:

- Cortisol, the stress hormone

- DHEA, an energizing hormone that declines with age, hence the decline in energy with age

- Aldosterone, the hormone that maintains salt and water balance in your body

Estrogen and testosterone, the primary sex hormones, are also produced in small amounts by the adrenals.

When you are stressed, the immediate fight-or-flight response is due to adrenaline. Soon cortisol kicks in for the long haul. It helps maintain blood pressure and heart function, slows the immune system's inflammatory response, helps balance the effects of insulin as it breaks down sugar for energy and helps regulate the metabolism of proteins, carbohydrates and fats.

Even though your body is designed to return to normal after stress, many of us are under continuous stress, keeping cortisol levels consistently high. This eventually leads to adrenal fatigue. Although this condition affects millions of people, conventional medical practitioners are still skeptical about its existence and won't treat adrenal weakness until the glands are in full collapse, called Addison's disease. Here is a typical example of low adrenal function:

Sarah admitted she had been a "slow starter" for the past two years. "I'm just tired all the time, even after I've slept a good eight or even nine hours," the 35-year-old ad agency account executive said. In fact, the fatigue had gotten so bad in recent months that she couldn't even keep herself awake in the evening in order to complete her day's work. She tried to keep herself up with cup after cup of strong black coffee but complained that it had almost no effect. She also snacked on chocolate bars and potato chips, saying it gave her some energy. "I'm a mess!" she complained to me.

I asked her to tell me about the stress she had been experiencing, and she threw up her hands. "Don't get me started. My life is nothing but deadlines, deadlines, and more deadlines," she sighed.

Everything Sarah said made it apparent to me that she had gone beyond stress into adrenal fatigue. When your adrenal glands can no longer meet the demands of unremitting stress, adrenal fatigue can lead to outright adrenal exhaustion. In rare cases, adrenal fatigue can also be caused by tuberculosis, fungal infection, amyloidosis, or cancer, so it's important to rule these out before you continue with treatment.

Symptoms of Adrenal Fatigue

Here are the general symptoms of adrenal exhaustion:

- Unexplained fatigue
- Difficulty getting up in the morning even after a sufficient amount of sleep
- A feeling of being overwhelmed
- General feeling of being run-down

- Difficulty bouncing back from illness
- Repeated infections
- Inability to let stressors go
- Craving for salty and sweet snacks
- Energy pickup after 6 p.m.
- General achiness
- Low blood sugar
- Low blood pressure
- Dizziness upon standing up suddenly (postural hypotension)
- Waking up in the early morning hours with anxiety

Testing

Take the Adrenal Stress Index laboratory test to discover if you are suffering from toxic stress. It involves a series of samples over the course of a day to measure your DHEA and cortisol levels.

Here are the DHEA normal ranges (saliva):

> Women ages 19–30: 29–781 mcg/dL
> Women ages 31–50: 12–379 mcg/dL
> Postmenopausal women: 30–260 mcg/dL

And the cortisol normal ranges:

> Morning: 4.3–22.4 mcg/dL
> Night: 3.1–16.7 mcg/dL

If your test results are outside the normal ranges, you are certainly suffering from stress overload, and the many ways of alleviating your stress (see Chapter 9) will give you relief. Normal is highly relative, and these scores are a bit deceptive. The important points are that DHEA diminishes with age and that cortisol should be higher in the morning than at night. The "normals" you deal with will be your own.

You might want to consider retaking the lab test for stress at the end of your eight-week Vibrant Health Plan to see how you are doing. Your results will be clearly explained in the report that accompanies your test results.

SELF-TEST FOR ADRENAL FATIGUE

Here's an excellent self-test for low adrenal function. You'll need a blood pressure cuff or monitor and a helper.

Lie on your back for at least five minutes. Then have your helper record your blood pressure.

Sit up quickly and have your blood pressure taken again.

Stand up quickly and take it again.

In people without adrenal dysfunction, the blood pressure will rise between 4 and 10 points with each measurement. If your blood pressure drops for either or both of the last two measurements, it's likely that you have adrenal exhaustion.

Medical Treatment

Cortef

Hydrocortisone (brand name Cortef) is a corticosteroid, also frequently prescribed for arthritis, anemia, severe allergies, lupus, multiple sclerosis, and a host of other conditions. I prescribe it in doses of 5–20 mg a day in divided doses, nowhere near the large doses that are usually in the form of prednisone, whose side effects are hard to distinguish from the symptoms: fatigue, joint pain, slow wound healing, increased susceptibility to infections and adrenal insufficiency. Even more serious side effects have been reported, including vision disturbances, confusion, euphoria and depression. The small doses, on the other hand, are safe and can be tapered down once the adrenals are working properly. I prefer the compounded *sustained-release* capsules over the commonly used Cortef, for a smoother, longer-lasting effect.

Natural Approaches

Vitamin C: Studies show that people with adrenal insufficiency excrete large amounts of vitamin C in their urine, so it's important to keep your supplementation levels high.

Cautions: If you experience diarrhea, adjust your dosage downward and then gradually build back up.

Dosage: Take up to 6 grams a day.

DHEA: DHEA can help bring down high cortisol levels. It may may convert excessively to estrogen (eg causing breast tenderness or water retention) or testosterone (masculinizing features). In those cases, I recommend 7-Keto DHEA, which is not diverted to the other hormones. While DHEA is a hormone, it can be purchased through the usual supplement suppliers.

Cautions: DHEA levels should be monitored since it can convert to other hormones with unwanted side effects. In cancer-susceptible women, DHEA many enhance the growth of abnormal cells.

Dosage: Most women need 5–25 mg daily. Your levels should be monitored evry four months or so.

Echinacea: Also known as purple coneflower, echinacea is a powerful immune system stimulator and has been shown to "wake up" exhausted adrenals. It's also helps you overcome the infections that often accompany adrenal imbalance.

Cautions: Take it in cycles of eight weeks on, one wek off to maintain its effectiveness. Echinacea stimulates the immune system, so you should not use it if you have an autoimmune disorder such as lupus or MS; AIDS or if you're HIV-positive.

Dosage: Take 325 to 600 mg of encapsulated freeze-dried Echinacea plant or 1,000–2,000 mg of dried Echinacea root three times a day.

Ginseng: Asian (panax), American (panax quinquefolium) and Siberian (eleutherococcus) ginseng are all helpful for adrenal exhaustion. Ginsengs are often referred to as "stress tonics" because they help tone the adrenal glands, normalize adrenal function and enhance your ability to resist the physiological effects of stress. Asian or Chinese ginseng (panax ginseng) is the strongest and may be too intense for some people.

Cautions: Take ginseng for three weeks, then stop for one week before resuming it. This way our body gets the biggest tonic effect. You can continue this pattern for up to two years.

Dosage: Take 100 mg of Asian ginseng twice a day using an extract standardized to 4% to 7% ginsenosides. For eleuthero, also known as Siberian ginseng, take 200 to 400 mg daily of an extract standardized to 1% eleutherosides.

Licorice root (*glycyrryza glabra*): Licorice is an adrenal stimulant, so think of a short course of licorice root as a natural jump-start for exhausted adrenal glands. It also manages hypoglycemia (low blood sugar) which often accompanies low adrenal function and chronic fatigue syndrome.

Cautions: Licorice can raise blood pressure or cause unusually high cortisol levels if used for too long. Women at risk for estrogen-senstive cancers should not use licorice nor should people with high blood pressure, kidney problems or abnormally low potassium levels.

Dosage: Take 200 to1,000 mg of glycyrrhizin extract (the active ingredient in licorice) daily for up to six weeks. Resume, if necessary, after a two-week break.

Pantothenic acid: Vitamin B_5 is known to support adrenal function and can be taken as part of a high potency vitamin B complex, which usually contains 10 to 50 mg daily.

Cautions: None at the recommended dose.

Dosage: Take 100 to 500 mg daily. I often prescribe 500 mg twice daily for a month or so, then reduce to once daily or 250 mg twice a day and eventually to 100 mg once a day to restore and support healthy adrenal function.

Adaptogens

Ashwaganda (*withania somnifera*): A traditional Ayurvedic medicine, ashwaganda can enhance the immune system, calm stress, and reduce levels of cortisol. It also enhances memory and mental acuity due to its antioxidant effects and ability to increase acetylcholine-receptor activity. On top of all this, it's an aphrodisiac! Ashwaganda can also increase thyroid hormone levels and basal body temperature. In a study on animals with arthritis, it proved better at reducing symptoms than hydrocortisone, suggesting that it has potent effects on adrenal hormone balance as well.

Cautions: None.

Dosage: Take 300 mg two to three times daily.

Reishi Mushroom (*Ganodermum Lucidum*): When I asked him about reishi mushroom, well-known herbalist and author Christopher Hobb replied: "I often take reishi myself and have experienced immediate calming and sleep-promoting effects. I have noticed an amazing feeling in my chest with some reishi extracts, as if my heart area has opened up. This unique effect, while not scientifically proven, is entirely enjoyable and often is accompanied by a feeling of immediate serenity." All I can say is, I'll have what he's having!

Rhodiola (*Rhodiola Rosea*): Modern science has confirmed that this revered ancient Chinese elixir can improve mood and energy, balance stress hormones, boost immunity, and improve concentration, especially in tired individuals. It can also raise serotonin levels, and encourage weight loss.
Cautions: There are no known side effects.
Dosage: Take 100 mg of a standardized product (2 percent rosavin and 1 percent salidroside) three times daily with meals.

Energy Balance Formula: This is my combination formula with three adaptogens—eleutherococcus senticosus, rhodiola, and reishi mushroom, plus tyrosine, TMG, B vitamins, and magnesium. A simple and effective treatment for adrenal fatigue, can keep you from crashing during the day while helping your adrenals to heal. (www.drcass.com)

Dietary Measures

Some of the most difficult aspects of adrenal insufficiency can be addressed easily through diet.

First, and most important, avoid stimulants of all kinds. This includes caffeine in coffee, teas and soft drinks and the biggest no-no of all, sugar. As much as you might think you need them to keep going, stimulants actually force your adrenal glands to work harder and become more exhausted. You want to give them a rest so they can recover.

Second, consider a low-glycemic diet (see Chapter 5), especially if you are prone to low blood sugar, as many sufferers of adrenal exhaustion are, with complex carbs in the form of fruits and vegetables.

Other Natural Treatments

You're already doing many of the things that will help bring adrenal function back into balance. Your exercise program is vital at this time because it will provide good stimulation for your adrenals.

Relaxation, meditation and yoga will also help restore the balance that extreme stress has disrupted.

Sarah's tests showed she had both low cortisol and low DHEA, signifying adrenal exhaustion. She took a stress-management course at the local wellness center. She also started taking the daily regimen of a multivitamin plus an extra 2 grams of vitamin C and 10 mg of DHEA. And, when she started to feel she was getting run-down or ill, she added echinacea. She also took my special adaptogenic Energy Balance Formula. After about four months, Sarah was looking and feeling much better. Her stamina had improved and, although her work situation itself had not changed, she was handling it far better.

CHRONIC FATIGUE AND FIBROMYALGIA

Have you suspected you have chronic fatigue syndrome (CFS, also called CFIDS) or fibromyalgia? Or have you been diagnosed with one of these debilitating conditions?

Do Sarah's story and the saga of adrenal exhaustion sound uncomfortably familiar to you?

It's not surprising if you do have chronic fatigue, because two-thirds of all chronic fatigue sufferers have adrenal imbalance.

Chronic fatigue and fibromyalgia have such similar symptoms and treatments that some argue they are the same, or variations of the same condition. Others suggest that long-term chronic fatigue may deteriorate into fibromyalgia. CFS is a relatively common condition affecting 500,000 Americans at any one time and twice as many women as men.

Symptoms

While both conditions are characterized by profound exhaustion and flu-like symptoms lasting for at least six months, sleep disturbances, muscle and joint pain, and headache, there are some differences between the two.

A diagnosis of CFIDS usually includes a chronic sore throat, headaches of a new type or of increased severity, tender lymph nodes, and feeling tired rather than invigorated after exercise. It often begins after a flu or other viral infection.

Fibromyalgia sufferers may experience intense body stiffness and joint pain, numbness or prickling in extremities, facial pain, abdominal discomfort, irritable bladder, chest pain, allergies, cognitive disorders, clumsiness, visual confusion, nausea, sensitivities to light, noise, odors and weather, and depression and anxiety. There are specific trigger points that are especially tender to the touch.

The most common symptoms are debilitating fatigue in CFS and chronic body pain and interrupted, unrefreshing sleep in fibromyalgia. But crossover symptoms are common, and there are a variety of other symptoms and markers astute practitioners look for in making a diagnosis. But unfortunately, as you suffer these symptoms, you may face the additional challenge of getting properly diagnosed.

Diagnosis

If you've suffered with these symptoms, you've probably gone from one doctor to another trying to find out what's wrong with you. Some of the more shortsighted members of the medical profession actually consider CFS and fibromyalgia to be "fad" diseases or psychosomatic illnesses! Both conditions are extremely difficult to diagnose and really require the help of a dedicated doctor who will spend the time necessary to confirm a diagnosis and devise a treatment plan for you. If you are exhausted to the point where it interferes with your life and paradoxically cannot sleep (and are not depressed), and the fatigue does not go away with a vacation, you probably have CFS. If you ache all over in addition to not being able to sleep, you have fibromyalgia as well.

You need to be tested for conditions such as hypothyroidism, adrenal exhaustion, lupus, Lyme disease, a variety of viruses including Epstein-Barr and cytomegalovirus, and rheumatoid arthritis. Intestinal yeast/candida is often present and needs to be treated, as well (see Chapter 14).

Here are some medical clues:

- Low blood pressure
- Oral temperatures under 97 degrees

- Slightly elevated oral temperatures, but less than 100 degrees
- Increased heart rate
- Unsteadiness on standing with eyes closed

These are some tests that may help your doctor reach a diagnosis:

- CBC with a Chem-20 panel
- Erythrocyte sedimentation rate (ESR), a marker of inflammation
- Urinalysis
- Antinuclear antibodies and rheumatoid factor
- Thyroid tests (TSH, T3, T4)
- Adrenal tests (a.m. and p.m. cortisol levels)
- Lyme disease titers
- HIV test
- Epstein-Barr, cytomegalovirus, and Coxsackie antibody titers

Possible Causes and Medical Treatment

The causes of these conditions are likely a combination of various factors. Likely infectious in origin, they could be caused by viruses ranging from herpes to Epstein-Barr and Coxsackie. There is also some evidence that both conditions might be caused by mycoplasma, a tiny microorganism that invades the entire system and shares characteristics of both bacteria and viruses. This can be determined only through growing a culture in a lab. Treatment lasts three months to a year, usually with several types of antibiotics. Heavy metal toxicity is often associated with CFS, and should be addressed as well (see Chapter 15).

Hormones

Many women with fibromyalgia are menopausal and postmenopausal, and their condition often improves with natural hormone replacement therapy (see Chapter 11). Measure your levels of thyroid, estrogen, progesterone, DHEA, and testosterone, and follow with appropriate replacement therapy.

Lifestyle

- Get eight to nine hours of sleep a night (which may require some sleep aids).

- Balance your hormones.

- Treat the underlying infections.

- Get proper nutritional support.

- Pace yourself and engage in only moderate exercise.

- Try some of the following: physical therapy, acupuncture, aquatic therapy, chiropractic, massage, self-hypnosis, tai chi, therapeutic touch, and yoga.

For excellent information on CFS and fibromyalgia, see Dr Jacob Teitelbaum's website, www.vitality101.com.

Natural Supplements to Treat CFS and Fibromyalgia

These are in addition to those for adrenal support

5-hydroxytryptophane (5-HTP): Lack of deep (stage 4) sleep may be one cause of the pain of fibromyalgia, and this may be due to low serotonin, the calming mood-elevating neurotransmitter. 5- HTP will help to raise levels of serotonin.
Cautions: Be sure to take a multi with vitamin B$_6$, required for 5-HTP's conversion to serotonin.
Dosage: 100–200 mg 30–60 minutes before bedtime.

B vitamins: High doses of B vitamins have been shown effective in relieving fatigue in people with both conditions. Adding TMG (trimethylglycine) to B-complex helps lower levels of hyomocysteine, which has been linked to fatigue.
Cautions: None known at recommended dosage.
Dosage: Take according to label directions.

Cetyl Myristoleate: This fatty acid is effective for the treatment of fibromyalgia and arthritis.
Cautions: None, except that it is quite expensive.

Dosage: Take three 1,500-mg softgels daily on an empty stomach.

Malic Acid: Through a complex biochemical reaction, malic acid, a fruit acid, helps reduce lactic acid, thus relieving muscle pain. It can be taken as magnesium malate, to provide magnesium, which is often low in CFIDS patients and is an excellent muscle relaxant. It is also found in Corvalen M, in combination with ribose.
Cautions: none
Dosage: 350 mg three times daily

Melatonin: Melatonin helps improve sleep patterns and relieve pain, making it an ideal supplement for chronic fatigue and fibromyalgia. This universal antioxidant has been proven to penetrate cell membranes and provide protection to all cells. It protects the central nervous system against injury, disease and aging.
Cautions: May cause excessive dreaming, headache, daytime sleepiness or irritability. Not recommended if you have rheumatoid arthritis.
Dosage: Take 3 mg before bedtime. A time-released version will prevent early morning awakening.

Padma Basic Herbal Formula: Padma Basic is an excellent and safe "cooling" or anti-inflammatory herbal formula from Tibet. It has an impressive amount of research to back up its use as an antioxidant, and has a role in enhancing circulation and immunity as well.
Cautions: Can cause rapid heart rate in sensitive individuals (similar to the effects of coffee).
Dosage: Take one tablet twice daily, increasing as needed.

Ribose (or, more properly, D-ribose): One of the building blocks of cellular energy or ATP is a form of sugar called ribose. Although it is found in small amounts in red meat, most of it is made in the body. Ribose is useful for treating fibromyalgia, where there is insufficient blood flow or oxygen supply, so you can't make enough ribose to generate energy. Combine ribose with L-carnitine and CoQ_{10} for a good boost in energy. This combination also also essential for heart muscle action, so helps combat heart failure.

Cautions: Diabetics taking medication need to monitor their insulin levels when taking it, since ribose can lower blood sugar.
Dosage: 1 teaspoon (5 gms) of powder twice daily. Can be taken in combination with magnesium and malic acid, available as Corvalen M.

SAMe (s-adenosylmethionine): Generally used as an antidepressant, it has also recently been shown to relieve joint pain that results from declining SAM-e levels as we age, leaving us vulnerable to arthritis and muscle pain, making it an effective treatment for CFS and fibromyalgia.
Cautions: Can cause irritability, anxiety, nausea and vomiting at high doses. SAM-e can trigger manic episodes in people with bipolar disorder.
Dosage: 400–1,600 mg daily.

Ginseng, echinacea and other therapies for adrenal exhaustion may also be helpful.

Valerian (*valeriana officianalis*): Valerian enhances GABA activity in the brain to produce a calming effect similar to that of Valium without the side effects. It reduces anxiety, tension, and insomnia. It is nonaddicting and has no next-morning hangover. I also prescribe it for those tapering off the Valium-type drugs (benzodiazepines) such as Klonopin (clonazepine), Xanax (alprazolam), and Ativan (lorazepam).

Be forewarned—its smell has been likened to old socks, so you'll probably be happiest taking it in capsule or tablet form.
Cautions. Valerian increases the effects of other sedative drugs, including muscle relaxants and antihistamines. It can interact negatively with alcohol, narcotics, and other psychotropic drugs.
Dose. To promote relaxation, take 50–100 mg two or three times a day. To help you sleep, take 100–400 mg 45 minutes before bedtime. Look for a standardized product with 0.8 percent valeric acid.

The adaptogens and other therapies for adrenal exhaustion may also be helpful in treating chronic fatigue syndrome or fibromyalgia.

Other Approaches

Myofascial Release is a highly specialized gentle stretching technique used by physical therapists to treat patients with a variety of soft tissue problems, and has been helpful in treating fibromyalgia.

Hot baths with added Epsom salts (magnesium sulfate) can help relieve muscle and joint pain, both because of the heat because magnesium is a natural muscle relaxant, well-absorbed through the skin. Swimming in a heated pool is also useful, due both to the warmth and the movement.

Acupuncture has been helpful to many people with chronic fatigue syndrome and fibromyalgia.

According to Mary Shomon, author of *Living Well with Chronic Fatigue Syndrome and Fibromyalgia* (Collins, 2004), "I talked to dozens of the nation's top CFS and fibromyalgia researchers, and one thing became clear: There are effective treatments, but they need to be carefully customized to each person. No one solution works for everyone, and anyone who suggests that is misleading. Ultimately, the best chance of remission or recovery is when you look at the potential conventional, holistic and alternative theories and solutions and, with a knowledgeable practitioner guiding you, choose the right mix of approaches for you." Her book and website are first-rate guides for anyone with these conditions and their families (www.cfsfibromyalgia.com).

13

BLOOD SUGAR IMBALANCES
From Metabolic Syndrome to Diabetes

"You've got a little sugar," the kindly family doctor told Kathleen's mother-in-law 50 years ago. "Not to worry. Cut back on the cakes and pies, and everything will be just fine."

It wasn't. Within 10 years, Kathleen's mother-in-law was dead of a grim series of strokes that left her increasingly debilitated until she finally gave up. Her many sons and daughters were only a little better off. Five more have died of complications of diabetes, and four others have the disease, with their side effects ranging from quintuple bypass surgery to amputations—and this generation has had the benefit of modern medicine.

The kindly family doctor meant well, and, to be fair to him, no one knew much better 50 years ago in the Philippines.

Diabetes isn't "just a little sugar," and blood sugars outside the normal range mean you need to take action. Right now. It's serious.

Type 2 diabetes has reached epidemic proportions in the United States, primarily because we are growing, literally, larger and larger and at younger and younger ages.

Once called "adult-onset diabetes," it is no longer a disease limited to adults. Children as young as 10 are being diagnosed with Type 2 diabetes, and they're condemned to a shorter, more painful life as a result.

In the not-too-distant past, the only diabetes we saw in children was juvenile-onset or Type 1 diabetes, in which the pancreas stops making insulin, requiring careful blood sugar monitoring and daily insulin shots. Now, poor diets and obesity are leading to a whole new generation of diabetics. Whatever the patient's age, most cases begin with a metabolic disorder referred to as metabolic syndrome, syndrome X or insulin resistance.

Jennifer, a 49-year-old housewife, was discouraged that she was unable to lose the extra pounds she'd accumulated in the past five years, particularly around her middle. She said her husband complained that she gets pretty cranky when they are on the road and late for a meal. She admitted, "I know I overeat. I just need it to help me feel OK," referring to her favorite foods: pasta, bread and sweet desserts. Her only vegetable was mashed potatoes with lots of gravy!

METABOLIC SYNDROME

Jennifer had the signs a relatively newly recognized condition called Metabolic Syndrome. Here are some of the symptoms:

- Mental and physical sluggishness

- Weight gain

- Difficulty losing weight

- Steady, slow escalation of blood pressure

- Slowly rising cholesterol and triglycerides

- Escalation of blood sugar

All of these symptoms are often written off as the aging process, but they don't need to be, and they're reversible.

The major factor in Metabolic Syndrome is insulin resistance. In their book *Metabolic Syndrome* (Wiley 2000), Jack Challem, Burton Berkson, M.D., and Melissa Diane Smith explain insulin resistance as "a diet-caused hormonal logjam that interferes with your body's ability to efficiently burn the food you eat." It is possible to be insulin resistant if you don't have Syndrome X. For the latest information, see Challem's new book, *Stop Prediabetes Now* (Wiley, 2007).

If you've been in the habit of consuming lots of high-sugar foods, including white flour, candy, cookies, baked goods and fruit juices, your blood sugar levels are probably bouncing around. As your blood sugar goes higher after you eat, more insulin is secreted to cope with the sugar. Insulin removes the sugar and stores it as fat and glycogen (a form of sugar that can be released later when it is needed). High-sugar foods cause insulin to spike rapidly and excessively, causing blood sugar levels to drop, resulting in feelings of weakness, light-headedness, and irritability. So you eat more of the same, and the vicious cycle goes on, as in Jennifer's case. Newer research indicates that this feeling may also be due to hyperglycemia, as you cylce from low to high and back down again.

Our diets high in sugar and refined carbohydrates and processed foods are causing us to literally overdose on two elements essential for human survival: glucose and insulin. Not only are you risking diabetes, but the excess glucose levels speed the aging process and set the stage for degenerative diseases through the production of destructive free radical oxygen molecules, often simply called *free radicals*. These are unstable molecules that damage cells and age them (aging is simply the accumulation of damaged cells). Add to this the advanced glycation end products (AGEs) produced by excess glucose, and you have a vastly speeded up aging process, setting the stage for all kinds of degenerative diseases: diabetes, heart disease, cancer, arthritis and Alzheimer's disease.

The good news: You can start to reverse the process, and you'll notice the difference within days.

Testing

You may have already done the simple finger prick blood sugar test, which led you to this section.

Your fasting blood sugars should be between 80 and 100 mg/dL. Above 110 can be normal if you've eaten in the past couple of hours. Even if you've eaten recently, your glucose should be below 180. A normal postprandial (after meal) level is between 70 and 140 mg/dL.

Below 70 is called hypoglycemia (see information later in this chapter).

If your test results show impaired glucose tolerance, you may want to ask your doctor for a glucose-tolerance test. You'll drink a special heavily sugared drink, and blood will be drawn over a period of time (two to six hours) to determine how well you are metabolizing the sugar. Fasting blood sugar levels outside the normal range are a warning that your ability to metabolize glucose is impaired. Insulin levels may also be elevated, with the normal range being 6–35 mcIU/ml. It should be less than 25. Another measure is hemoglobin A1c or glycosylated hemoglobin, which measures your average blood sugar over a 90-day period. Normal range is 4–5.9%.

Low blood sugars can also be caused by stress leading to adrenal fatigue after repeated demands on the adrenal glands for cortisol and adrenaline. These stimulating hormones result in feelings of anxiety and profound fatigue. For more information on adrenal exhaustion, read Chapter 12.

Jennifer's lab tests showed a fasting blood glucose at 125 mg/dL. Her blood pressure at 140/90 and a total cholesterol of 225, together with her weight gain, fatigue, and carb cravings, made her diagnosis of Metabolic Syndrome quite obvious.

The Nutrition and Exercise Factors

Improving your diet is the first step toward conquering Metabolic Syndrome (and its end stage, diabetes). We've said it many times, and it bears saying here again, with feeling: The typical American diet, heavy on sugar, refined carbohydrates and processed foods, is causing your health crisis. If you have not cleaned your kitchen of these health wreckers, put down this book and do it now.

If you are overweight, as are 90% of people with impaired blood sugar metabolism, it's essential that you begin to bring down your weight as soon as possible. Read Chapter 17 on ways to address weight problems. Weight management is not just a matter of "toughing it out" or eating lettuce (or any of the many fad diets). It's a lifestyle adjustment for the rest of your life. Your life will be a longer one than it would have been without these changes.

In addition to our recommendations in Chapter 17, adding lots of fiber to your diet is especially important in addressing blood sugar levels. Research published in the *New England Journal of Medicine* shows that people whose diets included 25 grams of soluble fiber and 25 grams of insoluble fiber lowered their blood glucose by 10% in just six weeks. Fiber also helps protect against heart disease and cancer.

That's a lot of fiber. It's about double the current recommendations of the American Dietetic Association. It means eating at least nine servings of fruits and vegetables a day plus oatmeal, whole grains, bran and dried beans. Read labels to determine if you're getting enough fiber. For a listing of the fiber content of common foods, go to www.fatfreekitchen.com/fiberlist.html. You can always add a tablespoon of ground flaxseeds or psyllium husks dissolved in a glass of water (or diluted juice) to increase dietary fiber.

Making these modest dietary changes and adding light exercise has been proven to lead to a 20% decrease in insulin resistance.

Remember Jennifer, whose 125 mg/dL fasting blood glucose put her at high risk for diabetes? Simply improving her diet by eliminating the doughnuts at her coffee break and her after-dinner desserts and adding a 15-minute walk every day before lunch dropped her fasting sugars to 100 mg/dL in three months. Her cholesterol also came down nicely.

If you've been diagnosed with Type 2 diabetes, your new nutrition plan will be the same and you can expect to achieve excellent results. Many diabetics have actually been able to discontinue prescription medications after improving their diets and adding exercise.

You're sure to have noticed that we highly recommend exercise. It's not just because exercise is a nice thing to do or it makes you look good. Both are true. But there are distinct physiological results of exercise that are dramatically demonstrated in people with insulin resistance.

Exercise increases the amount of muscle in the body and decreases body fat. Because muscle cells are effective in pairing up glucose and insulin, the more muscle you have, the better you are able to process carbohydrates.

If you eat well and exercise, your body will process the high-quality carbs more slowly, releasing sugars in a measured way. The additional muscle mass from your exercise program will give you the tools you need to process carbs into fuel for your cells.

Medical Treatment for Metabolic Syndrome

Metformin (Glucophage) lowers blood sugar in your system by slowing sugar production and absorption, helping your body respond to its own insulin. Many physicians now prescribe metformin as the first drug of choice for people with diabetes. Among its many benefits, metformin does not cause weight gain. However, it also has many side effects, including depleting various vitamins such as folic acid and B_{12}, essential for heart and brain function, resulting in elevated homocysteine levels. This is a serious risk factor for heart disease. As usual, it's far better to look beyond symptom relief (elevated blood sugar) with medication and go to natural means that address the root of the problem. For more details on blood-sugar lowering drugs, see my book, *Supplement Your Prescription* (Basic Health, 2008).

Natural Approaches

Here are some supplements that will help lower your blood sugar, increase your body's sensitivity to insulin, and can be excellent preventive measures. If you have been taking oral diabetic medications of any kind, do not stop taking them without consulting your doctor.

If you're already on oral diabetic medications, these may help them be more effective, thereby lowering your dose. You must monitor your glucose levels carefully and work in partnership with your doctor to ensure a healthy blood sugar balance.

Consider these:

Alpha lipoic acid (ALA): ALA reduces insulin resistance and improves your body's sensitivity to insulin, thus lowering blood glucose and insulin levels. ALA has been scientifically proven to increase glucose burning so your body has less demand for insulin. It also has an unknown mechanism to delivering glucose to cells by somehow bypassing the insulin delivery system. A potent antioxidant, it neutralizes disease-causing free radicals. ALA also increases cellular energy levels. It has been shown to reduce the incidence of macular degeneration and cataracts that often accompany diabetes.
Cautions: Higher doses can cause gastrointestinal upset.
Dosage: To prevent Metabolic Syndrome, take 100 mg daily along with other antioxidants such as Vitamins C and E. For Metabolic Syndrome and glucose intolerance, take 100–250 mg, daily in divided doses, with meals. Diabetics may take up to 600 mg daily under their doctor's supervision, since it may lower the required doses of their glucose-lowering medications.

Carnitine (L-carnitine): This amino acid helps your body burn glucose more efficiently, balancing your blood glucose levels. It's been shown to improve insulin sensitivity, protect against diabetic neuropathy, protects against heart disease and help in fat burning for efficient weight loss.

Cautions: Avoid taking carnitine after 3 p.m. because it may give you too much energy to be able to sleep well. Start with low dosages (500–1,000 mg) and build up slowly to prevent gastrointestinal upsets.

Dosage: Up to 2,000 mg twice daily. It's fairly expensive, about $4 a day at high dosages. It can be taken in powder form to minimize both the number of capsules, and the price.

Biotin: This water-soluble member of the vitamin B-complex family helps your body use glucose efficiently by enhancing your metabolism of carbohydrates. It works with insulin to increase the activity of glucokinase, an enzyme responsible for better glucose metabolism that is often low in people with diabetes. It's found in cooked egg yolk, most fish, liver, poultry, dairy products, beans and brewer's yeast and, of course, supplements.

Cautions: None known, but should not be taken in high doses by pregnant and nursing women.

Dosage: Take 1,000 mcg three to six times a day.

Chromium: Keeps glucose levels under control and manages blood sugar over the long-term, fights insulin resistance, helps with weight control. About 90% of American adults are deficient in chromium. It is available as both chromium picolinate and chromium nicotinate.

Cautions: Do not exceed 1,200 mcg daily. High doses have been associated with kidney and liver damage. Do not use it if you're pregnant or nursing.

Dosage: Take 500 mcg. twice a day.

Coenzyme Q_{10} (CoQ_{10}): CoQ_{10} is a potent antioxidant and cellular energy enhancer. It helps the insulin-producing cells work better and improves the metabolism of glucose. It's especially important if you are taking cholesterol-lowering drugs that dangerously deplete your body's stores of CoQ_{10}. Studies show CoQ_{10} supplementation can help liver, kidney and heart function.

Cautions: Taking CoQ_{10} late at night may cause insomnia. It may also cause mild gastrointestinal discomfort.

Dosage: 100–300 mg daily in divided doses. Also take up to 500 mg of quercetin twice a day.

Vitamin E: This antioxidant reduces free radical damage, increases insulin sen-

sitivity and prevents complications arising from inflammation. One study shows vitamin E supplementation increased the removal of glucose from the body by 47%. Vitamin E also works to reduce the risk of heart disease by stopping inflammation in the circulatory system. It is also essential to take along with your fish oil to prevent the latter's becoming oxidized in your body
Cautions: None.
Dosage: Take 400–1,200 IU daily.

Magnesium: This mineral lowers blood sugar, increases insulin sensitivity and helps your body cope better with stress. This last benefit is important because stress is known to aggravate diabetes. Magnesium deficiency, which is present in many people with diabetes, is believed to interrupt insulin activity. Magnesium also improves insulin's ability to transport glucose to cells, making it essential for anyone with high blood sugar.
Cautions: May cause diarrhea at high doses.
Dosage: Take 200–400 mg of magnesium up to three times a day. To increase absorption, be sure to get 30–50 mg of vitamin B_6. The most absorbable forms are magnesium aspartate, glycinate or citrate.

N-acetyl-L-cysteine (NAC): This antioxidant protects insulin producing cells from being damaged by free radicals. When taken in combination with vitamins B and C, it can partially neutralize excess in the blood, thereby helping to treat Metabolic Syndrome.
Cautions: None known.
Dosage: Take 500 mg a day on an empty stomach with 250 mg of vitamin B_1 and 1,500 mg of vitamin C twice daily or as tolerated.

Bilberry: The fruit of the bilberry bush has been shown to substantially reduce blood glucose levels as well as triglycerides or blood fats. It is also good for maintaining eye health.
Cautions: May cause blood thinning. Do not use if you are taking blood thinners like Coumadin.
Dosage: 80 mg twice a day.

Cinnamon: Studies show that cinnamon-yes, the normal type that tastes great sprinkled on baked apples—has a powerful blood-sugar lowering capacity. The credit goes to a polyphenol in cinnamon called MHCP, which acts just like insulin and helps transport glucose into the cells, lowering blood glucose by 20% within weeks.

Cautions: None.

Dosage: $1/2$ teaspoon a day or stir your tea with stick cinnamon (not the candy form).

Essential Fatty Acids (EFAs): We've mentioned essential fatty acids before. They are very important for people with diabetes, glucose intolerance and Metabolic Syndrome because they reduce inflammation with is a part of the syndrome and an element of heart disease.

Cautions: Since mercury is a concern in most fish, be certain of your source. Wild-caught fish are definitely safer. Look for a supplement that is derived from molecularly distilled fish body oil, and is marked mercury-free on the label.

Dosage: Add wild-caught salmon, mackerel, tuna or other fatty fish to your diet twice a week. Sprinkle a tablespoon of ground flaxseed over your salad, cereal or veggies every day. You can also take it supplement form. Look for a product that has at least 800 mg of EPA and 400 mg of DHA, the essential ingredients of fish oil. You'll probably need to take about 2–3 grams a day to get these levels.

Milk thistle (*silybum marianum*) and silymarin: Milk thistle and its active ingredient, silymarin, have been used for two millennia to treat liver-related disease. A properly functioning liver improve glucose control. A large human study shows silymarin dramatically improved patients with glucose intolerance and it's been shown to protect kidney cells from the toxic effects of excess glucose.

Cautions: None.

Dosage: Take 200 mg of a standardized product daily.

Fenugreek (*trigonella foenum-graecum*): Studies show these seeds can lower blood glucose and lower cholesterol, treating major symptoms of Metabolic Syndrome. It works best in people with mildly elevated blood sugars.

Cautions: At high dosages, can cause flatulence.

Dosage: Take 5–10 grams daily or buy it in bulk at an Indian grocery and mix in foods, tea or plain water. If the taste doesn't suit you, stir it with a cinnamon stick (not the candy type).

This may seem like a lot to tackle, but you can find supplement formulas on the market that contain combinations of these nutrients. See www.drcass.com for specific formulas.

HYPOGLYCEMIA (LOW BLOOD SUGAR)

This condition, related to diabetes, has sometimes been called *carbohydrate intolerance* because your insulin-releasing mechanism is impaired in a manner similar to diabetes. Hypoglycemia is usually the result of eating simple carbohydrates (i.e. sugar or white flour), which can trigger your pancreas to overreact and release too much insulin, thereby lowering blood sugar. When patients come to me complaining of anxiety, hypoglycemia is the first thing I look for.

These are symptoms of hypoglycemia:

• Fatigue, dizziness, shakiness, faintness

• Irritability, depression

• Weakness or cramps in feet and legs

• Numbness or tingling in hands, feet, or face

• Ringing in the ears

• Swollen feet or legs

• Tightness in chest

• Heart palpitations

• Anxiety, nightmares, panic attacks

• Night sweats

• Constant hunger

• Headaches and migraines

• Impaired memory and concentration

• Blurred vision

- Nasal congestion

- Abdominal cramps, loose stools, diarrhea

Subclinical (under-the-radar) hypoglycemia is difficult to diagnose because symptoms may be subtle and irregular, and tests can be within normal ranges.

Clinically, if your blood sugar drops below 70, you are considered hypoglycemic. A drop in blood sugar three or four hours after a meal is a sign of carbohydrate intolerance.

Standard Medical Treatment

The usual treatment when blood sugars fall dramatically is to add simple sugars in the form of sugar, fruit juice, soft drinks, candy or glucose tablets. While this will normalize blood sugars temporarily, it will only cause them to crash again in an hour or two unless you eat protein and complex carbohydrates with the sugar. If you've been diagnosed with diabetes, hypoglycemia may be a signal that your medications need to be adjusted. The sugar treatment is not recommended as a long-term way of treating hypoglycemia, but it can be useful in an emergency.

Natural Approach

The first and simplest way to treat hypoglycemia naturally is to balance your diet. Consuming a diet high in protein, slowly absorbed unrefined carbohydrates and moderate healthy fats is the way to keep those sugars balanced. Eat several small meals daily, beginning with breakfast. Avoid alcohol, caffeine and tobacco because they can trigger an episode.

Consider these supplements that can help to stabilize low blood sugar. Start with a multivitamin as your base.

Chromium and vitamin B_6: Chromium helps release stored sugars in the liver. Vitamin B_6, supports chromium's work and protects brain cells form excess glucose.
Cautions: None
Dosage: Take 200 mcg. of chromium with 100 mg of vitamin B_6.

Glutamine: As the most common amino acid found in muscle tissues, gluta-mine plays a vital part in the control of blood sugar. Glutamine is easily con-verted to glucose when blood sugar is low.

Cautions: None

Dosage: Take up to four 500 mg capsules daily with your regular supplements or add glutamine powder to a protein drink (without sugar). Best taken 30 minutes before a meal.

Hypoglycemia is not very difficult to control through diet and these simple supplements, but it's important to address the issue. It is a warning sign that you must address your carb intake or risk developing Type 2 diabetes. This is not to be confused with untreated hypoglycemia in a diabetic, which can be life-threatening.

STRESS MANAGEMENT

Managing your stress is an important part of your Vibrant Health Plan to bal-ance your blood sugar.

Now is a good time to read or re-read Chapter 9 on stress imbalances.

If you're not already doing so, make time for yourself every day. Meditate, take a stroll in the park or soothe yourself in a sudsy bath.

Jennifer's story had a happy ending. She joined a gym, where she alternated aerobics with weight training, discovered a whole new way of eating that she actually enjoyed and was thinking of running a marathon for her age group. She looked and felt better than she had in years. Her husband thanked me as well!

14

DIGESTION, DYSBIOSIS, AND FOOD ALLERGIES

Martha, a 33-year-old mother of two young children, described herself to me: "I'm a mess! I'm spacey, depressed, and nervous. I feel bloated after meals, like I'm pregnant." She was also sensitive to odors, such as newsprint, perfumes, and new fabric smells in stores. In addition, she had serious PMS and heavy periods.

Her combination of symptoms plus her history provided all the clues I needed. As a teenager, Martha was given tetracycline for two years to treat acne. Then she was on birth control pills for three years until she and Max were ready to start a family. After her second child was born, she began having bouts of vaginitis two, three, sometimes even four times a year. She also complained of recurring bladder infections and mentioned she had been diagnosed with endometriosis. I was sure she had systemic candida overgrowth, even without taking any tests. I did have her take a stool test, but rather than wait for the results, I began treatment right away.

How did Martha have all these medical problems, and what is candida?

THE FUNGUS AMONG US

Healthy women have a natural community of yeasts, primarily *Candida albicans,* that live in the warm, inner creases of the digestive tract, vagina, and skin.

(Men have yeast in their gastrointestinal tracts as well.) If you have a healthy immune system, these fungi interact symbiotically with your friendly intestinal bacteria such as *Lactobaccillus acidophilus* and *Bifidobacteria bifidum.*

When the friendly bacteria are eliminated, often through the use of antibiotics, the yeasts start growing out of control. They burrow into the gut wall, causing "leaks" in the protective barrier. Toxins and allergens, including undigested food particles, are allowed to enter the bloodstream. This is called "leaky gut syndrome." These leaks further compromise your immune system, leading to a long list of symptoms. Along with dysbiosis, we often see recurring vaginitis or endometriosis, depression, headaches, fatigue, interstitial cystitis, PMS, Crohn's disease, food allergies, chemical sensitivities, and possibly autoimmune diseases such as rheumatoid arthritis, lupus, asthma, psoriasis and more. Yeast is a great instigator and imitator of numerous conditions.

Some questions that come up: Does the yeast overgrowth actually *cause* these conditions or simply make them worse? Or are both conditions caused by some other underlying imbalance? We know these are complex conditions, and it may seem simplistic to paint such a broad picture of these little organisms.

Whoa! We can hear you asking now: How can fungi in the digestive tract, or even in the vagina, affect every part of the body from skin to bladder to lungs to joints to reproductive organs? When these toxins or antigens enter your bloodstream, they can travel anywhere in your body, adding to any imbalances you may already have. We're not saying that depression, acne, food sensitivities or rheumatoid arthritis are always caused by dysbiosis. However, there's sufficient research and evidence based on thousands of cases to indicate it can be a contributing factor to many of these conditions.

The late Dr. William Crook, who was a pioneer in this area, developed an extensive questionnaire to help determine if candida yeast overgrowth is an underlying cause of health problems. We'll reproduce a portion of it here.

ARE YOUR HEALTH PROBLEMS YEAST-CONNECTED?

If your answer to any question is "yes," circle the number in the right-hand column. When you've completed the questionnaire, add up the points. Your score will help you determine the possibility (or probability) that your health problems are yeast-related.

1. Have you taken repeated or prolonged courses of antibacterial drugs?   4

2. Have you had recurrent vaginal, prostate, or urinary tract infections?   3

3. Do you feel "sick all over," yet the cause hasn't been found?   2

4. Are you bothered by hormone disturbances, including PMS, menstrual irregularities, sexual dysfunction, sugar craving, low body temperature, or fatigue?   2

5. Are you unusually sensitive to tobacco smoke, perfumes, colognes, and other chemical odors?   2

6. Are you bothered by memory or concentration problems? Do you sometimes feel "spaced out"?   2

7. Have you taken prolonged courses of prednisone or other steroids; or have you taken birth control pills for more than three years?   2

8. Do some foods disagree with you or trigger your symptoms?   1

9. Do you suffer with constipation, diarrhea, bloating, or abdominal pain?   1

10. Does your skin itch, tingle, or burn; or is it unusually dry; or are you bothered by rashes?   1

Scoring: if your score is 9 or more, your health problems are probably yeast-connected. If your score is 12 or more, your health problems are almost certainly yeast-connected.

So how did you get this insidious problem? There are two major underlying causes of dysbiosis: prolonged or frequent use of antibiotics and a diet heavy in sugar and processed foods. The two work hand-in-hand, and each one makes the other worse. Other causes are prolonged use of steroid hormones or birth control pills, and stress.

The word *antibiotic* means anti-life. When you take antibiotics, they kill all the bacteria in your system, good and bad. That's great when you want to get rid of bacterial infections or ulcers or bacterial pneumonia. They're necessary and they're life-saving. However, in recent years, many people have demanded antibiotics every time they get a cold or flu. The truth is, antibiotics are useless against viral infections like these, and all they do is upset your balance over and over. And they make you susceptible to other problems. They also make future courses of antibiotics less effective and create antibiotic-resistant strains of bacteria. Finally, they underscore the need to replace those lost friendly bacteria as soon as you finish a course of antibiotics. (See "Natural Approaches" later in this chapter.)

When the good bacteria, necessary for digestion and a wide variety of body functions, are eliminated, they give the yeast normally present in your digestive tract an opportunity to grow wildly. If the balance is not restored, it can lead to persistent vaginitis, irritable bowel syndrome, and eventually to all the negative effects of leaky gut syndrome.

Worse yet, yeast overgrowth often leads to sugar cravings. Because sugar literally feeds the yeast and helps it grow even more, a diet loaded with sugar, refined flour, and processed foods promotes yeast growth, causing an even greater imbalance.

This is the most basic description of dysbiosis and how it affects your whole system. Symptoms of dysbiosis are elusive and can relate to numerous other conditions. Here's a partial list:

- Fatigue
- Depression or manic depression
- Numbness, burning, or tingling in your hands and feet
- Headaches
- Muscle aches
- Muscle weakness or paralysis
- Pain or swelling in joints
- Abdominal pain
- Bloating, belching, or intestinal gas
- Vaginal burning, itching, or discharge
- Endometriosis
- Infertility
- PMS
- Anxiety or crying fits
- Cold hands or feet, low body temperature
- Nasal congestion or postnasal drip
- Sensitivity to milk, wheat, corn, or other common foods

- Heartburn

- Psoriasis

- Dizziness, loss of balance

- Sore throat

- Foot, hair or body odor not relieved by washing

- Wheezing or shortness of breath

- Recurrent ear infections

FOOD ALLERGIES AND CHEMICAL SENSITIVITIES

Food allergies and chemical sensitivities are systemic overloads frequently found in women with yeast overgrowth. This does not mean that they are limited to dysbiosis sufferers, but these conditions often go together. At the same time, there are many women who have food and chemical sensitivities who don't have dysbiosis.

Many doctors think the term "allergy" should be limited to those conditions that can be diagnosed by allergy skin tests and sophisticated laboratory tests. The benchmark is an increase in IgE (immunoglobulin E), which often causes that familiar "histamine reaction:" sneezing, runny nose, stuffy head, eczema, dermatitis, hives, itching and watery, itchy eyes. Even life-threatening anaphylactic shock that often occurs in cases of extreme sensitivity to penicillin, stinging insects, shellfish and peanuts. Many people are allergic to feathers pet dander, and dusts and molds in the household.

Then there are food allergies. The Asthma and Allergy Foundation of America says 90% of all food allergies are caused by just eight foods: milk, soy, eggs, wheat, peanuts, tree nuts, fish and shellfish.

Women with dysbiosis or candida infections often develop an allergy or hypersensitivity to molds, tobacco smoke and common household cleaning chemicals. The standard treatment for allergies is to avoid substances to which you're allergic. It's not that easy with allergies associated with dysbiosis because your symptoms may be cycling through your entire system. Many people with food allergies and sensitivities do not show a positive allergy prick test, and these are often called "hidden" or "delayed-onset" allergies.

IgG (immunoglobulin G)–mediated allergic responses are measured by an

elevated IgG level in the blood. Besides the common reactions generally identified as allergic, these types of food and chemical sensitivities (to distinguish
them from the IgE-mediated allergies) can show up as fatigue, headaches, irritable bowel syndrome, sleep disturbance—in fact, almost anything you can
think of.

You often won't know that your symptoms are related to sensitivity until you
remove the offending substance, such as stopping consumption of wheat or
dairy, and the problem disappears, only to reappear when the you reintroduce
the substance. You can track down your hidden food sensitivities by using the
eating plan in this chapter. One type of allergic reaction results in the typical
sneezing, stuffy head symptoms we all know, but another type is much more
subtle and is caused by food allergies that may not produce symptoms until
hours or days later.

A common related problem is celiac disease (CD), a genetically based sensitivity to gluten, which is the protein component in wheat, barley, rye and oats.
CD often goes hand in hand with dysbiosis. You can test yourself by eliminating gluten-containing products and seeing how you feel. Full-blown celiac disease may be more readily recognized because of chronic intestinal symptoms.
However, I have had quite a few patients who had never before been diagnosed
with CD discover that they had the condition after they tested positively to the
antigliadin antibody (through a blood or saliva test). I have also seen many
people who realized within a few days of eliminating wheat (or corn or dairy
products) that the pain in their necks or the back stiffness or ringing in the ears
(or any symptom you can imagine) had disappeared. The pain then reappeared
a few days later when they reintroduced the food. Recent research shows that
gluten sensitivity can be a risk factor for developing Alzheimer's disease if you
don't eliminate the offending (gluten-containing) foods.

DIAGNOSING DYSBIOSIS

Many women with dysbiosis or yeast have found little medical help for their
conditions, despite numerous trips to various doctors. That is due, in part, to
the difficulty in diagnosing dysbiosis and, in part, to the general lack of understanding in the medical community. These poor women have been accused of
hysteria, hypochondria, and worse by doctors who simply don't know about
this elusive condition.

You're most likely going to need to recruit a doctor to help you in this search, because some of the necessary laboratory tests must be ordered by a physician (see Chapter 18 for help).

Here's what you can expect from a complete diagnostic workup:

- **A request for your complete medical history.** This should include not only your present complaints but also a detailed medical history, starting with infancy. You should write this down before your appointment.

- **Physical examination.** This should include a gynecological examination and examinations of your skin, eyes, heart and lungs, plus any other part of your body that is concerning you. Your doctor should really look at you. A good doctor recognizes that there are many signs of health problems. Bags under the eyes and/or a wrinkle across the nose may mean hidden food allergies.

- **Laboratory examination.** Tests, including the basic blood tests we discussed in Chapter 3, plus urine tests, x-rays and more complex laboratory studies such as a stool test (available through www.gdx.net) will likely rule out other causes for your problems. If all else is inconclusive, your doctor may order a complete gastrointestinal panel for anti-candida antibodies. Your lab exams should also include a stool examination to determine if you are suffering from parasites, which can produce some of the same symptoms as yeast or bacterial infections

Your doctor may or may not get a conclusive answer from all of this information, because there is no clear-cut test that will tell if you have systemic yeast overgrowth.

If you've had vaginitis four times or more in the past year, it is almost certain that you have systemic yeast overgrowth.

Another means of diagnosing systemic candida is to start on a treatment program that features a sugar- and yeast-free diet and prescription or nonprescription antifungal medications. If the symptoms clear up with this treatment program, then the culprit was yeast.

MEDICAL TREATMENT

There is no true standard medical treatment for dysbiosis. In fact, many doctors don't think systemic yeast overgrowth is possible except in those with terminal cancer or AIDS or other diseases in which the immune system has effectively ceased to function. The idea that someone with candidiasis could be walking around, more or less performing the tasks of daily life, is inconceivable to most of these doctors. You'll need to find one who is more open to current thinking.

Others may treat vaginitis over and over with short courses of prescription antifungals such as Diflucan, but they still refuse to consider the concept that your infection could be system wide. You may find a good match by searching the websites of the American Holistic Health Association, the American Holistic Medical Association, the American Association of Naturopathic Physicians, the American College for Advancement in Medicine, and the American Academy of Environmental Medicine.

Once you've found a doctor who will listen and determine a course of action with you, the plan will be similar to the natural approach.

Many doctors taking a natural approach will still will want to use prescription antifungal medications, perhaps for a long period of time. While there are serious side effects associated with these pharmaceuticals, sometimes the yeasts have been growing so wildly for so long that there is little alternative.

I always start with natural remedies, as you can, too, leaving the medication to the more difficult cases.

Here are some of the most commonly used prescription antifungals. You should be closely monitored for liver toxicity (i.e., monitor liver enzyme levels) while you are taking any of these drugs.

Diflucan (Fluconazole)

Diflucan (or fluconazole, its less expensive generic form) is the most commonly prescribed medication for short-term treatment for vaginitis. It's also used for long-term treatment of yeast overgrowth because it works throughout your system to penetrate tissues infested with candida microorganisms. It can be prescribed for four to eight weeks in difficult-to-treat candidiasis. Side effects include headaches, nausea, vomiting, abdominal pain, and diarrhea. The dosage usually tapers off after a few months, and a maintenance dose may be as low as one pill a week. These other two related drugs may be considered depending on your individual situation:

- Sporanox (itraconazole)
- Nizoral (ketoconazole)

Nystatin (Mycostatin)

Available in the United States since 1951, Nystatin is an effective and safe anti-fungal medication that works in a unique way to reestablish the strength of the intestinal walls, eliminating leaky gut syndrome. Nystatin is virtually free of side effects, with the exception of possible minor gastrointestinal upset. It is not absorbed into the bloodstream but remains in the gut to do its job there. At about 60 cents a pill, it is by far the cheapest of the prescription antifungals. Plus, patients rarely report die-off, a natural part of the detoxification process that produces flu-like symptoms when yeast organisms begin to die and release toxic wastes. The downside is that some strains of candida are resistant to Nystatin. Some doctors will start patients on Diflucan for a few weeks and then switch to Nystatin.

NATURAL APPROACHES

The heart and soul of treatment for systemic yeast overgrowth is dietary. Whether you choose to take prescription antifungals or natural remedies, you must eliminate sugar, yeast and processed foods from your diet for a few weeks, maybe indefinitely. If you don't combine diet with other treatment, the relief will be only temporary.

The anti-yeast eating plan is not easy, we'll be the first to acknowledge that. However, once you start feeling so much better, you'll find you're well rewarded for the sacrifices.

The plan involves eliminating sugar and yeast and foods you suspect may be related to your symptoms for at least three weeks. Then you'll gradually start reintroducing specific foods and recording your results.

This is a multistep process:

1. **Eliminate problem foods.** This is unquestionably the hardest part. You'll eliminate all sugar and all foods containing sugar, processed foods that often contain sugar and chemical additives, fruit and all yeast and fungi for the first three weeks.

2. **Control what you eat.** During the first three weeks, you can eat the following foods freely:
   - Low-carbohydrate vegetables (except mushrooms)
   - Lean cuts of beef, pork, and poultry
   - Fish

   You can cautiously eat the following:
   - Dried beans and peas
   - Potatoes (white and sweet)
   - Winter squash
   - Dairy products (except cheese). Yogurt may be especially beneficial.
   - Whole grains (not breads)

   You must completely avoid the following:
   - All sugars and sugar-based foods, including honey and maple syrup
   - All boxed and packaged foods
   - Fruit
   - Breads, pastries, and bakery goods
   - All cheeses
   - Condiments, sauces, and foods containing vinegar
   - Malt products
   - Processed and smoked meats
   - Mushrooms (Depending on your own case and tolerances, they may actually be beneficial because they are immune boosters.)
   - Melons
   - Dried and candied fruits
   - Leftovers (which may grow mold)
   - Fruit juices
   - Alcoholic beverages
   - Soft drinks (diet or regular)

   Remember, this is not a weight-control plan. While you are likely to lose some weight, your intention is to identify the foods that are contributing to your symptoms.

3. **Challenge.** No doubt you're feeling much better after the elimination phase of your eating plan. You'll start experimenting by eating a small portion of a suspect food. You can add in a piece of fruit and record your responses. Then, a day or two later, try some starch such as pasta. Challenge with only one food at a time and space each challenge by at least 24 hours, preferably more. This process will probably take several weeks, but you'll be developing a list of your hidden food allergies that will serve you well.

4. **Reassess.** If you're still having symptoms, you'll need to dig deeper into the sources of your food sensitivities. Progressively eliminate some of the basic foods that were allowed during the elimination phase and see if you get results. You may also have parasites or a viral problem such as Epstein-Barr virus, cytomegalovirus, or others.

5. **Maintain.** Once you've discovered your triggers, you can lighten up a bit on the program. You can fine-tune your personal program because you know what works. If you challenged yourself on fruit and passed the test, add moderate amounts back into your diet, but probably not more than three or four pieces per week. You might even be able to tolerate bread a couple of times a week without triggering symptoms.

As your digestive system heals, you will be able to tolerate more foods.

Natural Supplements

Find more details on these natural supplements, including recommended doses and cautions, in the Appendix.

Caprylic acid: This naturally occurring fatty acid is a powerful antifungal that has been around for 40 years. It is easily absorbed and virtually side-effect free.
Cautions: None at the recommended dosage. If the symptoms of die-off become too uncomfortable, reduce the dosage for a few days and then build back up.
Dosage: 1,000 to 2,000 mg three times a day with meals. It will probably take two to or three months at this dosage to entirely clear your system. Look for an enteric-coated version so the caprylic acid can have the maximum effect by slowing releasing throughout the digestive tract.

Citrus seed or grapefruit seed extract: This broad-spectrum natural antibiotic kills a wide variety of pathogens that may be upsetting your system. It works much like caprylic acid and Nystatin in stopping the growth of candida in the digestive tract. It has the additional benefit of being effective against parasites.

Cautions: Unless the label specifically states otherwise, most citrus seed extracts are made from grapefruit. Since GSE can interfere with the effectiveness of some prescription medications, check with your doctor first if you're on medication.

Dosage: Take 500 mg three times a day.

Garlic: This pungent herb has been used for centuries to treat all sorts of ills, including candida overgrowth. It apparently works by strengthening the immune system by helping white blood cells eliminate toxic challengers. There has been a great deal of research on the multitude of health benefits on odorless aged garlic extract.

Cautions: None, even at high dose.

Dosage: 400–600 mg twice a day. You can get capsules to avoid garlic breath, or you can eat it fresh in virtually unlimited quantities.

Olive leaf extract: The active ingredient in olive leaf extract, oleo oleuropin, attacks all types of microbes, ranging from viruses to fungi and yeast organisms. These all help improve immune system function. Olive leaf extract may cause die-off, the flu-like symptoms that take place when the yeast starts to die and release their toxins. If you feel worse for a few days after beginning to take olive leaf, hang in there and know it's working! It should pass within a few days.

Cautions: None, even at high dosages.

Dosage: Take up to 1,000 mg per day, with meals if you prefer.

Oregano oil: Wild-crafted oregano oil is well known in the Mediterranean world for its ability to destroy fungi and yeasts, bacteria, worms, parasites and viruses. In *The Cure is in the Cupboard* (Knowledge House, 1997), Cass Ingram, D.O., describes the health benefits of oregano, proclaiming that "wild oregano is a veritable natural mineral treasure-house, containing a density of minerals that would rival virtually any food."

Cautions: You may smell like a pizza

Dosage: 5 drops of oil twice daily or 500 mg capsule twice daily

Probiotics: These natural friendly bacteria restore the perfect balance to your digestive system. The basic probiotic formula will contain *Lactobaccillus acidophilus* and *Bifidium bacterium,* but many formulas will contain additional beneficial organism. While probiotics are not the most powerful agents for knocking out yeast, they are a foundational part of any treatment plan for dysbiosis. They also help keep your digestive tract flora balanced once the yeast has been eliminated.

Cautions: None at recommended dosage.

Dosage: Get your probiotics in supplement form, follow package directions since there are so many types. They come in capsules, tablets, beverages and powders. The best probiotics are enteric coated, which means they can survive the passage through the stomach so they can do their work in the intestines. Look for a product that has at least one billion bacteria per serving. There are some that claim very high content (up to 60 billion organisms), but most of those don't survive sitting on the shelf. Refrigerated products are best because more of the bacteria will survive.

These treatments may cause die-off, the flu-like symptoms that take place when the yeasts start to die and release their toxins. If you feel worse for a few days after beginning to take olive leaf, hang in there and know it's working! It should pass within a few days.

It took several months for Martha to get back on track, but then it had taken a while for her to get as sick as she was. She started taking a combination formula containing caprylic acid, oregano oil, grapeseed extract and probiotics at the same time she began the elimination eating plan. "I had a few rough days with the die-off, but I lowered the dose for a week and then stepped it back up without a problem," she said. When she did the food challenge, Martha was surprised to find her sensitivity to yeast (as in bread) was very high and that she was allergic to wheat and dairy products, so she stopped eating them for a while longer.

Six months after our first visit, Martha came to see me, and she looked like a different woman! She had lost weight and gained muscle by working out regularly with weights. Her brain fog had cleared, much to her relief. Her skin was clear, her step was brisk, and she proudly announced that she had not had a vaginal infection since she started the program. She was able to tolerate wheat and dairy once or twice weekly, as well. She was one of those who didn't have true celiac disease but a wheat intolerance caused by the yeast.

The keys to candida treatment are balancing diet, taking supplements including probiotics and minimizing stress and the other factors that are known to cause it. Once you have had candida, you must be ever watchful for its recurrence. The best prevention is to continue taking probiotics daily or every other day and avoid sugar and other offending foods.

15

ENVIRONMENTAL TOXIN IMBALANCES

When Rachel Carson wrote *The Silent Spring* in 1962, the world began to awaken to the dangers pesticides pose to the future of the human race. Now, more than 40 years later, many laws have been enacted to protect land, air, and water. Yet we are still continuously exposed to a chemical soup originating from industrial pollution, from so-called safe additives to food and from our very homes. These toxins have had long-range effects on our health, and they will continue to do so as long as we live in an industrialized society.

A frightening 2004 British study shows that the blood of virtually every person tested contained a cocktail of potentially deadly chemicals. In one of the most comprehensive studies of long-term effects of toxic chemicals to date, the study looked at 77 chemicals known to be "very persistent" in the environment and to accumulate in the human body. The most alarming finding was that 99% of those tested had residues of the pesticide DDT in their blood, despite the fact that it was banned decades ago.

As a result of this study, in 2007, the European Union began to require registration, safety evaluation, and authorization of thousands of everyday chemicals. Unfortunately, the United States lags far behind this progressive approach.

We've all heard of the "epidemic" proportions of breast cancer among women in San Francisco's suburban Marin County. There was a similar epidemic of leukemia among children in northern Nevada. Then there's the now-famous tale of the real-life Erin Brockovich and the multitude of illnesses suffered by the residents of Hinckley, California, because of contamination by the nearby Pacific Gas and Electric power plant.

Every day, every single one of us is bombarded by chemicals. Even if you live in a pristine mountain wilderness, toxins drift on the air currents from factories hundreds of miles away. Even if you filter all your drinking water, you can absorb toxins through your bathing water. Even if you eat exclusively organic food, the soil where it is grown could be contaminated by pesticides applied there decades ago and you'd never know.

If you live in an older house, you may have lead pipes contaminating your water and layers of lead paint under the newer latex. You may have asbestos insulation and mold problems.

If you live in a newer house, carpet and furniture will release toxic gasses for some months after installation, as will glue from fiberboard laminates. Naturally occurring radon gas could also be making you and your family sick.

Regardless of where you live, you're being exposed to flame-retardant chemicals used in everyday products like televisions, cars and even baby clothes. You may also be subject to carbon monoxide fumes if your house is too well insulated and you use an unvented open-flame heating system such as gas logs (they need a good chimney). You're almost certainly getting pesticide residues on fruits and vegetables you buy unless you grow your own or you can afford to buy organic products.

Then, of course, if you really love fish, especially the fatty fish we recommend for those crucial essential fatty acids, you're increasing your risk of toxic metal overload because fatty fish are known to concentrate these toxins in their tissues.

This isn't meant to scare you. It's meant to alert you to the dangers that are around and the measures you can take to keep yourself safe. It's a wake-up call to us all, and together we can navigate the minefield of toxins that surround us every day so we can recover our health.

The human body has an amazing ability to handle these types of attacks. When our immune systems are healthy, we are usually capable of neutralizing and rejecting bad guys, whether they come in the form of viruses, bacteria, yeasts, industrial chemicals, pesticides or even heavy metals.

However, if the body absorbs small amounts of these toxins over a period of years, the toxins can actually reach a critical mass and impair the immune system and symptoms can erupt, seemingly out of nowhere.

Even a low-level exposure to toxins can make some people sick because of a genetic malfunction that interferes with neutralizing enzymes. Others are simply sensitive to toxins, perhaps because they are very young or very old or because of health factors including smoking, drinking, diet, exercise and any health problems.

Toxic chemicals can get into your body through inhalation, through penetration of skin, or through your digestive tract. If you're pregnant or nursing, some can even cross the placenta, affecting unborn babies, and others can contaminate breast milk.

A recent study of newborn babies showed high levels of a variety of toxic chemicals in cord blood, 287 out of 400 that were tested for, indicating that they had been passed to the baby through the placenta. Of these, 180 cause cancer in humans or animals, 217 are toxic to the brain or nervous system, and 208 cause birth defects or abnormal development in animals. Scientists refer to the presence of such toxins in the newborn as "body burden." This is particularly alarming since babies are so vulnerable at this stage. (For the full report, go to http://www.ewg.org/reports/bodyburden2/.)

Once the toxins get into your body, they do their damage in a number of ways. Several types of toxins target the liver and kidneys, the organs that filter impurities from the body. Some chemicals and minerals migrate to fat and bone tissue where they can be released later. For example, lead is stored in bones and can be released during pregnancy, when you begin drawing on calcium stored in bone tissue.

These are the worst environmental toxins and how you can be exposed to them:

Mercury. This highly toxic mineral can be found in dental fillings, paints, tattoo dyes, ceramics, thermometers and electrical relays. Miners and workers in the manufacture of fungicides, thermometers and thermostats are at high risk of mercury toxicity. Symptoms include tremors, memory loss, loss of appetite and weakness. The main dietary source is fish, including shellfish. As our waters become more polluted, more fish contain mercury and the larger the fish the higher the mercury content. Note: Many people have chosen to remove mercury amalgam fillings from their teeth. If you decide to do this, be sure to seek out a dentist who is skilled at this procedure. Improper removal can increase your exposure to mercury vapors, and make matters even worse.

Lead. One of the most common toxins, lead can be found in water, paint, cigarettes, cosmetics, some pesticides, and foods such as meats, garden fruits, and grains. At highest risk of lead toxicity are workers in factories that manufacture or recycle batteries. It's also found in printing ink, gasoline, and some types of fertilizer. Lead is often deposited in bones, adrenal and thyroid glands, the brain, and the liver. Note: If you have an old house with lead paint, do not try to sand or remove the paint. Scraping can actually create lead dust and increase the risk. You'll either need to paint over it or have it professionally removed.

Aluminum. Used in the process of purifying water, aluminum is also found in large amounts in everyday household items ranging from cookware to cans. It's in antiperspirants, antacids, buffered aspirin and even some nasal sprays and toothpastes. Some research suggests long-term exposure to aluminum may be a factor in Alzheimer's disease. Symptoms of aluminum toxicity include memory loss, learning difficulty, loss of coordination and headaches. One of the few products that can extract aluminum is modified citrus pectin taken orally (Pectasol).

Asbestos. This fine, fiber-like mineral was widely used in construction, brake pads, fireproofing materials and chalkboards until it was proved to cause cancer and was banned in 1989. It can cause a wide variety of lung problems, lung cancer and a type of abdominal cancer called mesothelioma. Note: Do not attempt to remove asbestos-based building materials. Sometimes it is best to do nothing about asbestos that has been in place for a long time. Removal must be done professionally.

Benzene. This chemical is used in the production of deodorant, oven cleaner, soap and perfume. It's a component of paints, pesticides, asphalt, gasoline and jet fuel. It can contaminate groundwater and surface-water supplies and pollute air through automobile exhaust, manufacturing processes and cigarette smoke. Officially, benzene is considered hazardous only to the two million workers who are exposed to benzene in their jobs.

Formaldehyde. This chemical is used in the manufacture of many construction materials, including particle board, fiberboard, building insulation and plywood. The formaldehyde gas can be released by these products for several years after they are manufactured and installed. While the EPA says formaldehyde is a possible carcinogen, only industrial workers are considered at risk. Manufactured (mobile) homes are a particularly common source of this pollution and cause health problems to their inhabitants. This has been an issue in the Katrina victims forced to live in mobile homes that had not yet *outgassed* or fully released their formaldehyde content.

Radon. This is a colorless, odorless gas that is naturally present in the earth's crust and released into the air through radioactive decay. Certain areas of the United States have higher emissions of radon than others. The only way to tell if your house has a high radon level is to test for it. Test kits are available at most home supply stores. Long-term exposure to radon can cause lung cancer. Fortunately, a simple ventilation kit can correct the problem inexpensively.

Carbon monoxide. This common poisonous gas is released into the air whenever fuel, wood or tobacco products are burned. Heavy rush-hour traffic can produce high levels of carbon monoxide. Dangerous and potentially lethal levels can build up in poorly ventilated enclosed spaces because of exhaust fumes of faulty heating devices. Carbon monoxide poisoning can cause headaches, nausea and dizziness. At high levels, it can cause respiratory failure and death. Carbon monoxide detectors are efficient, inexpensive, and easy to install in your home.

Organophosphates. These residues of pesticides and insecticides present hazards for casual gardeners, farm workers, pest-control workers, landscapers and veterinarians. These toxic chemicals are usually absorbed through the skin. They can remain toxic for several days after they are applied to crops. Toxic effects can range from extreme fatigue to skin irritations, nausea, depression, breathing problems, seizures and coma.

SYMPTOMS

Symptoms of environmental toxin overload are wide and varied. You might experience something as simple as an apparent allergic reaction with sniffling, runny nose, sneezing, and watering eyes.

People who work in poorly ventilated buildings with high levels of airborne toxins re-circulating through the ventilation system may develop the flu-like symptoms called sick building syndrome.

Here's a list of the most common symptoms of chronic environmental poisoning:

- Cough
- Headache
- Nose and eye irritation
- Diarrhea
- Dizziness
- Blurred vision
- Loss of appetite
- Anxiety
- Memory loss

- Anemia
- Drowsiness
- Tingling in extremities
- Aching in muscles and joints
- High blood pressure
- Difficulty concentrating
- Fatigue
- Shaky hands
- Loss of coordination

These are symptoms in advanced cases:

- Depression
- Weakness
- Difficulty breathing

- Kidney failure
- Vertigo
- Learning disorders

Also note: Symptoms may disappear or diminish when you're not around the toxins, for example, over the weekend when you're not at the office or when you're away from home on vacation.

Once these toxins get a foothold in your body, they can open the door to other problems, including endometriosis, infertility, birth defects, heart disease, brain damage, respiratory problems and many types of cancer, particularly lung, breast and skin cancers.

Samantha has always loved older homes. In fact, at the age of 26, she started a business restoring old houses. Ten years later, the business was an enormous success with clients waiting in line, but Samantha simply didn't have the energy to keep up with the workload. "I feel like I have the flu all the time," she told me.

She also complained of headaches, a chronic cough, and dizziness when she climbed up on a ladder. "I really got scared and decided to come to see you when I noticed my hands were shaking uncontrollably," she told me.

It could have been any number of conditions, and it might have taken longer to diagnose Samantha's problems had I not asked what she did for a living. I ordered tests that led to her diagnosis: she was overloaded with lead and formaldehyde!

DIAGNOSIS

As you may have already discovered, it's difficult for a doctor to diagnose chronic environmental poisoning. The symptoms sound a lot like those of thyroid imbalance, chronic fatigue syndrome, fibromyalgia, sex hormone imbalance or depression. Most often, doctors have told these people that they were "stressed, and just needed to take it easy."

The first thing you'll need to do is compile a detailed personal history. This means not just your medical history but an accounting of anywhere you have lived or worked or played where you might have been exposed to environmental pollutants of any kind.

Here are some questions to get you started:

- Where have you lived?

- Did you live near a dump?

- Did you live near a paper mill or other type of factory?

- Did you live in an old house?

- Did you restore or renovate properties?

- Where have you worked?

- Have you worked in a factory that manufactured anything from fabrics to batteries to chemicals of any kind?

- Have you worked as a gardener, landscaper, or greenkeeper?

- Are you a dentist, or have you worked in a dental office?

- Have you worked in construction?

- Have you worked in a bar or in a place where you were exposed to large amounts of tobacco smoke?

- Do you have a long commute in heavy traffic?

- Do you eat a lot of larger fish such as swordfish and tuna?

While the answers to these questions may not give you an absolute diagnosis, they may begin to point the way to the source of your problem.

Tests

To start, get a good mineral toxicity testing kit. This test on a piece of your hair should reveal levels of toxic minerals including aluminum, antimony, arsenic, bismuth, cadmium, lead, mercury, nickel and tin. If you find toxic levels of any of these metals, we recommend you work with your doctor to further explore the problem. Your doctor will probably want to get laboratory analyses of your blood, urine and fatty tissues. On the other hand, most doctors do not address these issues, and you may have to find a specialist who does.

STANDARD MEDICAL TREATMENT

Your treatment will depend on what toxic substances are causing your problems. Treatments definitely should be individualized depending on your medical condition and the way in which you were exposed.

If you and your doctor have confirmed the diagnosis, the advice of an expert in poisoning should be enlisted. Most parts of the country have regional poison centers and medical toxicologists for added expertise.

Toxic metals, including lead are treated by specific oral, intramuscular or intravenous drugs. They bind with the metals in the blood by a process called *chelation* and are eliminated in the urine. Chelation is also effective in treating lead, mercury, aluminum, iron and arsenic poisoning, with a complex program of specific binding agents used for each type of poisoning.

Follow-up laboratory testing continues until your blood levels have returned to normal.

Clearly, a major priority in this method of treatment would be to remove you from the source of contamination and to remove the source of contamination from the place where you were exposed. This can be extremely difficult in some cases and fairly simple in others.

NATURAL APPROACHES

If you have been diagnosed with chronic environmental toxin poisoning, you must undergo medical treatment. However, there are many natural approaches that will assist in the detoxification process and promote your body's natural ability to detoxify.

Detoxifying Agents

These natural substances are clinically proved to assist with your detoxification.

Chlorella: This algae is rich in essential nutrients. It helps with detoxification, by binding with heavy metals in the colon and helping excrete them from the body. It's also been shown to be helpful in detoxifying from lead, mercury and chemical exposure.

Cautions: None.

Dosage: Take up to 9 grams a day, building up slowly to avoid diarrhea.

Modified Citrus Pectin: PectaSol® Chelation Complex™ is a patented blend of Modified Citrus Pectin (MCP) and an Alginate® complex, clinically shown to chemically bind heavy metals and other environmental pollutants. (www.drcass.com)

Cautions: None.

Dosage: As a dietary supplement, take 3 capsules twice daily on an empty stomach. Daily maintenance dose: For long-term maintenance take 2 capsules daily.

MSM (methylsulfonylmethane): This naturally-occurring compound contributes sulfur to make the amino acids glutathione, methionine, cysteine, and NAC, all essential for detoxification.

Cautions: None known.

Dosage: Take up to 3 grams (3,000 mg) daily.

Rutin: This plant extract is a free-radical scavenger with abilities to chelate excess iron.

Cautions: None known.

Dosage: Take $1/4$ teaspoon in powder form up to three times a day mixed in water or juice.

Antioxidants

It is very important that you keep your antioxidant levels high to keep out all sorts of toxins.

Alpha lipoic acid (ALA): This potent free radical scavenger has been shown to detoxify minerals and help revitalize the strength of other antioxidants. Some studies suggest ALA might help reduce lead and cadmium contamination.
Cautions: Higher doses can cause gastrointestinal upset.
Dosage: Take up to 600 mg of ALA daily.

Vitamin C: Research shows it can help reduce harmful effects of aluminum, lead, copper and radiation.
Cautions: If you experience diarrhea at high doses, back off your dosage and slowly build back up.
Dosage: Take up to 6,000 mg a day for detox. You can take higher dosages as tolerated.

Vitamin E: Helps strengthen lungs against inhaled pollutants.
Cautions: None.
Dosage: Take up to 2,000 IU daily with meals if you are suffering from poisoning.

Glutathione: Healthy levels of this powerful antioxidant have been shown to strengthen your body against heavy metals toxins and enhance your immune function. It has been used to treat lead, mercury, arsenic and cadmium poisoning.
Cautions: Do not use if you have kidney or liver disease.
Dosage: This is best taken as a liposomal oral liquid or a transdermal (skin) cream. See www.drcass.com for details.

Lactoferrin: This protein binds to iron, so it can be helpful in iron overloading.
Cautions: None.
Dosage: Take one 300 mg capsule daily.

Selenium and zinc: Essential to immune function, deficient amounts of these antioxidants leads to a compromised immune system.
Cautions: None at the recommended dosage.
Dosage: Take one 30 mg capsule of zinc and one 200 mcg. capsule of selenium daily.

Protective Agents

Milk thistle (*silybum marianum*): The active ingredient in milk thistle, silymarin, prevents liver damage and protect the kidneys, pancreas and other organs during a detoxification process. It is shown to be very helpful in speeding up detoxification and helping the liver regenerate after the process is complete.
Cautions: None
Dosage: Take up to 650 mg daily.

SAM-e (S-adenosylmethionine): Also called the liver's supernutrient, SAM-e can help protect your liver from destructive effects of chemicals and can help a damaged liver regenerate. It's been shown to be effective in protective against damage from toxic chemicals, cadmium and lead.
Cautions: High doses may lead to irritability, anxiety, insomnia, nausea or vomiting. Do not take if you are taking prescription antidepressants, without medical supervision.
Dosage: Take 800 mg daily and add B-complex for best absorption.

Even though it took almost a year, Samantha's case had a positive outcome. After undergoing eight treatments of chelation therapy, she was able to get the lead out of her tissues. The formaldehyde was a little more difficult, but on a careful program that included chlorella, glutathione, modified citrus pectin and milk thistle, she was back on the job with appropriate protective gear— and feeling great.

PREVENTION

Unquestionably, the best means of dealing with environmental toxins is to avoid them whenever possible.

Here are some preventive steps:

• Talk to your state environmental department to determine if your house is located in an area known for radon contamination. Have a radon test conducted if you are at risk.

- If you are removing paint from the inside or outside of your house, have it tested for lead content. Painting over old lead-based paint may be better than removing it. Sanding can release lead particles into the air.

- When you're using hazardous products, particularly insecticides and pesticides, follow the directions meticulously. Wear protective clothing, including a mask, and eye protection. Better yet, don't use them at all! There are many environmentally friendly and non-toxic options.

- Keep children and pets off lawns or gardens that have been treated with pesticides or herbicides. Stay indoors with windows closed when trees are being sprayed in your neighborhood. It's a good idea to leave outdoor shoes at the door and wear only specific indoor shoes to avoid tracking toxic substances inside.

- Use nontoxic cleaning products and insecticides in your house.

- Never use chemical pesticides on your houseplants.

- In buildings, be alert to chemical odors that may be emitted by paints, pesticides, new carpets or office machines. Check ventilation in your office to be sure it meets standards.

- Certain houseplants can remove impurities from the air, among them spider plants. Find more in *How to Grow Fresh Air* by B.C. Wolverton (Penguin, 1997)

- Avoid walking, running, or bicycling on streets where there is heavy traffic. Your higher breathing rate when you exercise will increase your intake of carbon monoxide and other toxins.

- Install a carbon monoxide detector in your home.

- If you are on a weight-management program, be aware that your body metabolizes fat for energy and if toxins have accumulated in fat tissue, toxins can be released as weight comes off. Your weight-management program should target gradual reduction so that your system does not become flooded with a sudden release of toxins stored in fat.

- Peel produce and consider buying organic whenever possible.

- Wash all fruits and vegetables with a mixture of hydrogen peroxide and vinegar to help cut toxic residues.

- Here's a useful tip from both Nan Fuchs and Ann-Louise Gittleman for removing pesticide residue from produce:

- Soak produce in a bath of 1 teaspoon of Clorox (no substitutes) to a gallon of water for specified length of time. Then soak in clear water for 10 minutes. Rinse and dry.

  ○ Leafy green vegetables—15 minutes

  ○ Root and fibrous vegetables—30 minutes

  ○ Thin-skinned fruits such as berries, plums, and peaches—30 minutes

  ○ Thick-skinned fruits such as citrus, bananas, and apples—20 minutes

  ○ Poultry, meat, eggs—20 minutes

  The process not only kills microorganisms but keeps the produce fresh longer.

- See dentists who do not use mercury amalgam and other toxic materials (www.holisticmed.com/dental/dental.res).

- Eat fish that are low on the food chain (i.e., the smaller ones that have not accumulated as much relative mercury as the larger ones that are higher up the food chain).

- Use nontoxic cosmetics because they are absorbed through the skin.

- Last, but far from least, remember that a healthy diet and supplementation program will help keep your immune system strong, your liver healthy, and your body at optimal readiness to fight off toxins.

16

MUSCULOSKELETAL PAIN
Headaches, Arthritis, and Osteoporosis

Headaches, arthritis, and osteoporosis take a toll on our comfort and sense of well-being and lead to limitations in our ability to function fully. When the bones and muscles that support you become imbalanced, the imbalances can show up as back pain, joint pain, carpal tunnel syndrome, pinched nerves or headaches. Then aging bring on the threat of osteoporosis, the thinning of bones.

Fortunately, you're not a helpless victim of musculoskeletal problems. While there are no quick fixes, there are many natural ways to address your pain, find relief and even, in many cases, end the pain. Narcotic pain medications and dramatic surgeries with their risks and side effects are rarely necessary, and they may even cause more pain than they cure.

There are some specialties outside of mainstream medicine that can often provide the solution to musculoskeletal problems. Among them are osteopathy, chiropractic, acupuncture, acupressure and massage. We'll discuss each of them in depth.

Let's start by looking at each condition separately, because each has its unique characteristics and treatment.

HEADACHES

The major types of headaches are tension or muscular headaches and migraine or vascular headaches. Sometimes the difference between tension headaches and migraines is very subtle.

Tension Headaches

If you've suffered from chronic headaches that haven't responded to drug therapy, you may be surprised to learn that almost all tension headaches come from muscle tension in your neck, shoulders and upper back. The tension usually comes from stress, from poor posture and occasionally from an injury. These headaches often occur late in the day and have at least two of the following symptoms:

- Pressing or tightening on both sides of the head
- Aching or squeezing sensation in the forehead, temples or back of the head
- Mild, moderate or even severe pain that begins gradually
- Usually not made worse by physical activity
- Occasionally, nausea or vomiting
- Light or sound sensitivity, but usually not both

Here's a typical headache-inducing scenario:

Your job promotes poor posture, whether you're bending over a drill press, hunched over a computer terminal or driving all day.

While you're doing this, your back is curved forward, shoulders rolled in, and chin jutted out. At home, you're curled up watching TV or reading while lying down.

Then you go to bed and sleep hunched over in the fetal position.

This cycle of poor posture trains your muscles to adapt to abnormal positioning, stretching out your back muscles, curling your shoulder muscles, straining your neck muscles and constricting your chest.

Continual strain on neck, shoulder, and upper-back muscles actually causes microscopic tears in the muscles. Your body responds by knotting the muscles to prevent tearing, causing them to spasm. More tearing takes place during the spasms, and over time, scar tissue forms over those tiny tears, locking the spasms in place.

The tension in your neck, shoulders, and upper back actually blocks the flow of blood to the back of your head, just like stepping on a turned-on garden hose. The tightness irritates nerves in the back of your head and neck and the headache starts.

Standard Medical Treatment

Most people with tension headaches use over-the-counter (OTC) medications such as aspirin, acetaminophen, naproxen, ibuprofen and other nonsteroidal anti-inflammatories (NSAIDs). But even OTC medications can have serious side effects, including sudden gastrointestinal bleeding and kidney damage. In addition, repeated use of these pain relievers can actually cause occasional headaches to become chronic.

Many doctors will prescribe prescription pain relievers and muscle relaxants for severe tension headaches. These have little lasting effect because they treat the symptoms and not the cause.

For extreme pain not eased by pain relievers, doctors sometimes prescribe antidepressants, anticonvulsants and beta-blockers, all medications that have serious side effects ranging from weight gain and sexual dysfunction to liver damage and memory loss.

Natural Approaches

Hands-on remedies are very effective in treating tension headaches. Most back pain will resolve with these methods as well. Even migraines will often also respond:

Chiropractic. A good chiropractor will be able to help relieve structural imbalances and muscular knots that are causing your headaches (and backaches). It may take several sessions, and you should be prepared to do some homework in the form of exercises and stretching.

Osteopathy. Osteopaths are traditionally trained medical doctors who are also trained in osteopathic manipulation. They can apply specific corrective forces to relieve joint restrictions and misalignments.

Massage therapy. This relaxing therapy can relieve tension before it piles up and can help correct postural problems as well. It's great in conjunction with chiropractic or osteopathy. There are also various forms of deep-tissue massage, such as Rolfing, which breaks up scar tissues that bind muscles and ligaments. It can be somewhat painful at the time, but ultimately, it can relieve your chronic pain.

Acupuncture. Using the principles of ancient Chinese medicine, an acupuncturist will observe your pulses, your eyes and even your tongue. Very fine needles are then inserted into specific places, opening blocked energy flow through unseen energy channels called "meridians." This often provides long-term relief for the tension that was causing the pain. The process is nearly painless. In fact, most people report a slight numbing sensation when the needles are inserted. To learn more about acupuncture and find a practitioner near you, go to www.acupuncture.com.

Acupressure. Acupressure uses the same basic structure as acupuncture, but without the needles. In fact, most people can perform acupressure on themselves. See Chapter 7 for specific instructions on acupressure to relieve neck and shoulder stress. Combining the acupressure application with deep breathing will increase its effectiveness.

Supplements. Any of the stress-relieving supplements in Chapter 9 will help to relax your muscles as well, especially magnesium and valerian.

Migraine Headaches

Migraine headaches are a serious problem affecting 28 million Americans, mostly women. These debilitating, throbbing, one-sided headaches are often unstoppable. They are commonly preceded by flashing lights or other visual disturbances and are accompanied by severe light sensitivity, nausea, and vomiting. My migraine patients describe themselves as lying curled up in a quiet, dark bedroom, ice packs on their necks, missing work, unable to take care of their families and in sheer misery.

Women sufferers far outnumber men, likely because of the hormonal influences. Sometimes sufferers can power through the headaches with the help of an anti-inflammatory or pain pill, or even avert them with potent drugs, but these medications unfortunately also have serious side effects.

Migraine headaches can be caused by a wide variety of factors, including stress, food sensitivities, and blood sugar, hormonal and musculoskeletal imbalances. There is research suggesting that low serotonin levels may contribute to migraines as well.

Well-known migraine triggers such as cheese, red wine, chocolate, eggs, mustard and smoked and processed meats also sap the body of the essential brain chemicals serotonin and noradrenaline. Avoiding these foods often can help prevent or at least diminish the frequency of migraines.

Caffeine withdrawal can also trigger migraines. If you drink more than two or three cups of coffee a day, consider this as a possible source of your pain and gradually reduce your caffeine intake as you switch to decaf or better yet, herbal teas.

Medical Treatment

There are numerous drugs on the market to stop migraines once they begin. Among them are the triptans such as Imitrex, Zomig, Maxalt and Migranal. However, there are serious side effects associated with them, including sudden heart problems, chest pain, severe allergic reactions, dizziness and drowsiness. They are not always effective, either.

Preventive therapy for migraine sufferers can include tricyclic antidepressants, blood pressure-reducing drugs, and anti-seizure mediations, all with their lists of side effects.

Natural Approaches for Migraines

Butterbur Root Extract: The softgel tablets have been shown in several studies to cut migraine frequency in half.
Cautions: None known.
Dosage: Take 50 mg three times a day for one month and then decrease to two times daily.

Coenzyme Q_{10}: Coenzyme Q_{10} has been shown to prevent migraines in a large number of patients. It has many other benefits, as well, including enhancing energy and well-being.
Cautions: None.

Dosage: Take 150–300 mg daily.

Feverfew: One of the most effective herbs for migraine prevention is feverfew. It may take up to three months to prevent migraines, so stick with it!
Cautions: May decrease blood-clotting ability, so it should not be taken with anti-coagulant drugs. It should not be used by pregnant women because it can cause uterine contractions.
Dosage: Take 250 mg. every morning. Look for a preparation standardized to 4% parthenolide.

5-Hydroxytryptophane (5-HTP): The serotonin-enhancing amino acid 5-HTP will help in migraine prevention.
Cautions: In rare cases and at very high doeses, 5-HTP can cause nausea, anxiety and agitation. For some sensitive individuals, it can cause anxiety at normal levels as well. Do not take 5-HTP with SSRIs except under medical guidance. While generally safe to combine, there is a risk of serotonin syndrome which inc ludes nausea, sweating, headache and a rise in blood pressure. If that occurs, stop taking this supplement.
Dosage: Take 100–300 mg daily, in divided doses. If it makes you drowsy, take it all at bedtime..

Magnesium: Intravenous magnesium administered in a doctor's office can stop a migraine in progress. Supplementation can also help raise serotonin levels, which are often low in migraine sufferers.
Cautions: Excessive magnesium acts as a laxative and may cause diarrhea. Use chelated forms like magnesium aspartate, glycinate or citrate. Magnesium has (rarely) been associated with drops in blood sugar.
Dosage: Take 500–1,000 mg daily for migraine prevention.

Riboflavin: With long-term use, B_2 helped reduce frequency of migraine attacks in 68% of those who took it.
Cautions: None.
Dosage: Take 200–400 mg daily.

Acupuncture

Acupuncture is an effective way of balancing serotonin production and has been shown in studies to reduce migraine severity by nearly 40%. For further details, look under "Tension Headaches."

ARTHRITIS AND BACK PAIN

Joint pain is the most common source of chronic pain and can result from trauma (such as a car accident), bone-weakening diseases like osteoporosis, repetitive motion, poor posture, foot problems that spiral upward throughout your frame, lack of physical activity and even the constant pull of gravity on bones and muscles as we age. There are two main types of arthritis: osteoarthritis and rheumatoid arthritis. Sometimes called degenerative arthritis, osteoarthritis is associated with the aging process and injuries. Rheumatoid arthritis is an autoimmune disease that can affect anyone of any age and affects multiple joints pn both sides of the body. Both types are painful and can be quite disabling.

Osteoarthritis and Back Pain

Osteoarthritis is the result of natural wear and tear on any joints, including the spine. Back pain is often caused by the deterioration of joints and of the disks or cartilage cushioning between spinal joints. However, it can be caused by misalignment of the spine, in which case chiropractic or osteopathic adjustments may be helpful. Many cases of back pain are caused by stresses on the muscles and ligaments that support the spine. An inactive lifestyle and excess weight can contribute to joint and muscle strain in the back or in other joints.

Rheumatoid Arthritis

Rheumatoid arthritis is an autoimmune condition in which your body is making antibodies to its own tissue, in this case, your joints. Women are much more likely to have rheumatoid arthritis than men. In fact, the likelihood of arthritis increases steadily from the time of your first period through menopause. Some women with arthritis notice their symptoms improve during pregnancy, confirming that the high levels of estrogen and progesterone during pregnancy can reduce inflammation in the body. This is why natural hormone replacement may offer relief. For more information on natural hormone replacement, please read Chapter 11.

Research also shows that people with arthritis have abnormally low daytime levels of melatonin. The so-called sleep hormone actually has far-ranging influences in your body, including regulation of sex hormones, balancing of body temperature, stimulation of immune system, and control of inflammation.

Sustained stress leading to toxic stress causes high levels of the stress hormone cortisol, eventually leading to adrenal exhaustion. Cortisol is not necessarily a bad guy. It actually helps you manage stress when it's working right. When cortisol levels begin to swing and become too low, you'll have higher levels of inflammatory compounds called cytokines, leading to more joint inflammation.

If your symptoms are worse at night or early in the morning, your cortisol levels may have dropped too low. This makes you more susceptible to pain and inflammation than at other times of the day when cortisol levels are naturally higher. Doctors have been using low doses of cortisol to relieve arthritis inflammation for more than 25 years.

Deficiencies of the adrenal hormone DHEA (dehydroepiandrosterone) contribute to bone breakdown that is also a part of chronic joint problems. You might gain some insight by reading about adrenal imbalances in Chapter 12.

Standard Medical Treatment

Doctors usually initially treat arthritis pain with over-the-counter remedies like aspirin, naproxen, or ibuprofen. These may provide some pain relief and may even reduce inflammation, but long-term use of even simple OTC drugs like these can have serious side effects that include sudden potentially life-threatening bleeding in the stomach.

The second line of defense against osteoarthritis pain is a class of fairly new nonsteroidal anti-inflammatory drugs called COX-2 inhibitors. The best known of these is Celebrex (celecoxib). Two other popular Cox-2 inhibitors, Vioxx and Bextra, were withdrawn from the market after studies showed it increased the risk of heart attack and stroke. These drugs do actually slow the production of the COX-2 inflammatory enzyme and relieve arthritis pain, but at a heavy price. Celebrex has been connected with sudden, and sometimes fatal, gastrointestinal bleeding.

Other medical treatments for arthritis pain include arthroscopic surgery and joint replacements. Arthroscopic surgery has come under fire as a "placebo" surgery, but it has been known to be effective to remove ragged edges from deteriorating cartilage and small, loose fragments from within joints.

Partial and total joint replacements are major surgeries with all the accompanying risks of surgery. They require a long recovery and rehabilitation period and they will fail after 10 to 20 years, simply because of wear and tear.

In the past few years, many doctors have begun to address long-term joint pain with injections of hyaluronic acid, a natural component of connective tissues that helps to cushion and lubricate joints. While these injections need to be renewed every 6 to 12 months, they are relatively painless, work quickly and have almost no side effects. They are far less expensive than surgery (about $700 a treatment, which most insurance companies will cover) when they work, but they are not effective for everyone.

Doctors often treat back pain with transcutaneous electrical nerve stimulation (TENS) units intended to block pain. Effective and side-effect free, they "fool" your body into not feeling the pain.

Another common treatment is with injections of pain-relieving steroids such as hydrocortisone into the joint. They need to be used sparingly, because more frequent use can have long-term negative effects, including elevated blood sugar, immune suppression, ulcers, cataracts and severe arthritis of the hip.

Prolotherapy is another treatment, consisting of injecting a sugar solution into an unstable joint. This will stimulate the proliferation of new ligament tissue in areas where it has become weak. The treatment is useful for many different types of musculoskeletal pain, including arthritis, back pain, neck pain, fibromyalgia, sports injuries, unresolved whiplash injuries, carpal tunnel syndrome, chronic tendinitis, degenerated or herniated disks, sciatica and partially torn tendons, ligaments and cartilage. See www.prolotherapy.com for details.

Natural Approaches

The goal of these approaches is to treat the cause of the pain. For osteoarthritis, you want to increase cartilage production. For rheumatoid arthritis, you need to address inflammation. Natural replacement of both progesterone and estrogen may give you the relief you are seeking. Supplementation with DHEA and melatonin may also be helpful, so they're included here.

Here are a few supplements that are effective in treating joint pain:

Ginger, turmeric and holy basil: These natural COX-2 inhibitors reduce inflammation and relieve arthritis pain with virtually no side effects. Studies show they work as well as Celebrex, without the risks. In fact, ginger is so safe it is recommended to relieve morning sickness in pregnant women.
Cautions: None.
Dosage: Take 100 mg of each herb daily. There are combination supplements available.

Glucosamine sulfate: This amino acid compound is one of the most widely used supplements in the U.S. Glucosamine has been shown to stimulate connective tissue and encourage it to repair itself. It has been shown to give cartilage the material it needs to repair damage from injuries and aging. Glucosamine sulfate does not work quickly like ibuprofen or aspirin. Expect to see effects in about eight weeks. It works best when taken with essential fatty acids and vitamins C and E.
Cautions: Do not use glucosamine if you are allergic to shellfish.
Dosage: Take 750 mg twice a day.

Chondroitin sulfate: Chondroitin, derived from shark cartilage, is often paired with glucosamine to provide additional building blocks for cartilage repair. It also slows free radical attack and stimulates blood flow to joints.
Cautions: None known.
Dosage: Take 600 mg twice a day.

MSM: Methylsulfonylmethane, a sulfur based compound, helps repair cartilage, rebuild collagen and stop inflammation, stiffness and pain. It has been shown to be very effective in relieving back pain. Research shows that people with arthritis have about two-thirds less sulfur in their cartilage than healthy people, and MSM delivers this mineral right where you need it. You'll often find it combined with glucosamine.
Cautions: None known.

Dosage: Up to 6 grams daily. You'll have to experiment to see what combination works best and relieves pain most effectively for you.

SAMe: S-adenosylmethionine, a natural antidepressant, has recently been proven to be at least as effective as NSAIDS like Celebrex at relieving osteoarthritis pain, swelling and stiffness. Research shows that your body's natural SAMe levels drop off as you age, leaving you open to arthritic changes and muscle pain.
Cautions: High doses may lead to irritability, anxiety, insomnia or nausea. In people with bipolar disorder, SAM-e may trigger a manic episode, so they should be monitored carefully.
Dosage: 200 mg of SAM-e once or twice daily, between meals, increasing gradually to a maximum of 1,600 mg a day, if needed.

Melatonin: Melatonin is in itself an anti-inflammatory nutrient that can be used for osteoarthritis and also helps increase the effectiveness of other remedies.
Cautions: Not recommended for rheumatoid arthritis, since some evidence suggests, however, that melatonin may worsen it .
Dosage: Take 3 to 10 mg before bedtime.

DHEA: Dehydroepiandrosterone has been called the "fountain of youth" hormone, not only for its effects on sex hormones, but for the way it can help you move like a younger woman. Manufactured by the adrenal glands, levels decline with age.
You will need to test your levels to determine the correct dose. (See Chapter 11.)
Dosage: Between 5 and 25 mg daily

Mind over Matter

Another approach is that of Dr. John Sarno, author of *Mind Over Back Pain* (Berkley 1999). His premise is that by dealing with suppressed emotions, you can relieve pain even when there is actual physical pathology. He has had a remarkable success rate and, to his credit, has taught his technique to the many of his patients. They continue to use it successfully if and when they experience pain, no longer needing to have the doc to "do it" for them. It's a refreshing change!

An Ounce of Prevention

You're probably reading this because you already have musculoskeletal pain. But it's never too late to develop habits that will improve your joint health.

Regular exercise is at the top of the list. Even if it is painful, keep moving. If you have knee, hip or back pain that prevents you from walking, consider an exercise bike. Be sure to do lots of stretching and warm-ups before each session and do an equally thorough cool-down. Ice packs can help ease swelling after a workout.

Good posture at all times is also important for joint and muscle health. This means you must insist on an ergonomic chair and keyboard at work, maintain proper posture while driving and take it upon yourself to have good posture at home. The best sleeping posture is on your back with a pillow under your bent knees or on your side with knees bent at a right angle with a pillow between your knees to keep pressure off your spine.

Massage, acupuncture and acupressure are all helpful in relieving joint pain.

OSTEOPOROSIS

Women constitute 80% of those affected with osteoporosis. This gradual loss of bone mass begins with the decline of hormones around age 40. By menopause, bone density can diminish rapidly.

Unless there are fractures, osteoporosis has no symptoms, although loss of height can be an indicator. Osteopenia (bone thinning) is considered an early warning of osteoporosis, with considerable loss of bone mass that stops short of osteoporosis.

Here are the risk factors for osteoporosis:

- Being female

- Thin or small frame

- Family history of osteoporosis

- Postmenopausal, including surgical menopause (hysterectomy)

- History of anorexia or bulimia
- Prolonged use of steroid medications
- Prolonged absence of menstrual periods after puberty
- Low-calcium, low-magnesium diet
- Lack of exercise
- Smoking
- Excessive alcohol use
- Excessive caffeine use

Keeping bones strong throughout your life is essential in preventing osteoporosis. Recent studies show that women who are athletic or highly physically active as teenagers have a significantly lower risk of osteoporosis as they age. On the other hand, overexercising can eat up the minerals your body needs to have strong bones.

We all need to think of osteoporosis as a life-and-death matter. The worst part of osteoporosis is that many of us have no idea it's happening until a bone breaks. Most of us know about the elderly woman's fear of a fractured hip, for good reason. About 300,000 women with osteoporosis break a hip each year. One in five of them dies within a year, and half are never able to live independently again.

If you've been diagnosed with osteopenia or even with osteoporosis, don't lose heart. There are many ways you can strengthen your bones.

Standard Medical Treatment

Most doctors want perimenopausal women to have a baseline bone density scan, a noninvasive x-ray-like test called a DEXA scan. It measures density of bone, usually in your hip, forearm and spine. Your results will probably be given to you in the form of a T-score that compares you to other healthy, young, adult women.

Bisphosphonates

If you've tested in the lower ranges, your doctor will most likely strongly urge

WHAT YOUR T-SCORE MEANS

Higher than −1: Your bone mass is close to average for a healthy, young, adult woman.

Between −1 and −2.5: Your bone mass is lower than normal, and your fracture risk is approximately twice as high as for the average woman. You have osteopenia or preosteoporosis.

Less than −2.5: Your bone mass is very low and your risk of fractures is approximately three times higher than for the average woman. You have osteoporosis.

Most doctors will want you to be on hormone replacement therapy if you have any loss of bone mass at all. They'll usually recommend you begin taking supplemental calcium, but that's only one-third of the story. Unless you're taking vitamin D and magnesium and other minerals, you won't be able to absorb the calcium.

you to take one of the newer medications reputed to prevent and treat osteoporosis. Many doctors are even pushing these potentially dangerous substances on women with normal bone density as a "preventive measure." Known as bisphosphonates, these drugs are commonly known as Fosamax, Skelid, Aredia, Didronel, Actonel and Zometa. They work by decreasing bone breakdown, with a net increase of bone mineral density and a reduced risk of fractures. They do this by binding to calcium in bones, making it more resistant to breakdown by osteoclasts. The big downside to these drugs is that by binding so closely to the bones, they slow the ability of the bones to heal themselves and can actually cause them to become more fragile in time. They have also been linked to a severe condition called *jaw necrosis,* where the jaw bone disintegrates.

Tamoxifen and Raloxifene

From a class of drugs known as selective estrogen receptor modulators, tamoxifen and raloxifene are often given to women who have been treated for breast cancer, to prevent a recurrence of the disease. Both have been found to improve bone density in these women, so raloxifene in particular is frequently prescribed for women with osteoporosis. Of course there is a little matter of a serious side effect: blood clots. We recommend against them.

Natural Approaches

Your most potent weapon against osteoporosis is supplementation with calcium, magnesium, boron, vitamin D, vitamin K, strontium, and soy. Adding a Chinese formula called *Osteophase* has also been very successful at preventing osteoporosis. Not far behind, are natural hormone replacement and weight-bearing exercise.

Natural Hormone Replacement Therapy

For women in perimenopause or menopause, natural hormone replacement therapy has a positive effect on bone health. Our bones have special receptors for estrogen. Not only can natural hormone replacement with both estrogen and progesterone stop bone loss, there is some evidence it can actually help rebuild lost bone mass. Estrogen helps prevent osteoporosis by decreasing the action of the osteoclasts or bone-dissolving cells. Progesterone stimulates the osteoblasts, which actually produce the bone cells. This makes progesterone the hormone of choice for bone health. See Chapter 11 on hormones for more information.

Exercise

Dozens of studies show that any exercise you do while standing on your feet will strengthen your bones. Walking, running, hiking, playing tennis, playing golf and dancing are all weight bearing exercise. You get the idea. It doesn't include swimming or cycling, although these are great for your heart.

In addition, weight-bearing exercise means weight training. No, that doesn't mean you have to become a bodybuilder. It means you should have a simple routine three or four times a week with hand weights and ankle weights or resistance bands. These tools are inexpensive and you can store them easily under your bed or in the coat closet. Take them out and spend five minutes on curls while you're waiting for the pasta water to boil or do some leg strengtheners while you're talking on the phone.

Supplements

Strontium: Not to be confused with the radioactive isotope strontium 90, a 2004 *New England Journal of Medicine* article showed that strontium combined with calcium markedly increased bone density.

Cautions: Take at least 700 mg of calcium a day (but separately) to balance the strontium (i.e., take more calcium than strontium).

Dosage: Take 340 mg twice a day between meals.

Calcium, magnesium, boron and vitamin D: These supplements are essential to bone growth and bone strength. They should be a part of every woman's life from puberty on.

Cautions: None at these dosages.

Dosage: If you're under 50, you need at least 1,200 mg of calcium, 800 IU of vitamin D, 400 mg of magnesium daily and 2 mg of boron. If you're over 50, you should be taking 1,500 mg of calcium along with the magnesium and D. You'll find many combination formulas that contain the precise mixture you need. You'll do best with a total mineral formula that will help strengthen bones by supplementing *all* of the 13 or more minerals in bones.

Soy products: These mild plant estrogens have been study-proven to improve bone density due to the presence of two active ingredients: genistein and daidzen. You can get soy in many foods ranging from tofu to miso to prepared veggie burgers. You can also get soy isoflavones in supplement form.

Cautions: Soy products should not be used by women with estrogen sensitivity, especially those who have had breast, ovarian or cervical cancer.

Dosage: Eat a serving of soy-based foods a day or include up to 200 mg of soy isoflavones in supplement form.

Vitamin K: This vitamin present in green leafy vegetable has been shown to reduce the risk of fractures in women and even improves the bone-building abilities of your natural proteins. It has been shown to improve bone density in women with osteoporosis.

Cautions: Vitamin K thins blood, so do not take it if you are using blood thinners like Coumadin.

Dosage: Up to 10 mg a day.

Osteophase: This specialized herbal formula from China has been shown to be excellent for restoring bone health in many women, as seen in improved DEXA scans. (www.drcass.com)

Cautions: None known.

Dosage: 4–6 capsules daily.

You can order a bone resorption wellness test that measures the bone turnover marker deoxypyridinoline (DPD), which is released into the circulation during the process of bone resorption. It can help you track the results of your therapeutic program.

3

ESSENTIAL INFORMATION FOR YOUR JOURNEY BACK TO HEALTH

17

MANAGING
YOUR WEIGHT

Never before in history have so many Americans been overweight, and never before in history have we been so concerned about our weight.

Many of us have obsessed about our weight since our early teens. At any gathering of women, it's bound to be a focal point of conversation. Everyone agrees MaryAnn looks great because she's just shed 44 pounds on an extreme low carb diet. Libby attributes her new figure to the South Beach diet. Kate became a vegetarian because her blood type is "A." Sue has been to Weight Watchers. Sarah is bemoaning her genetic misfortune because her dedicated, almost fanatical exercise and diet regimen has done nothing to slow the steady spread of her hips. Annie did it all with pills and coffee and looks gaunt and a little wrinkled, but she says that's better than looking puffy.

There's a new Weight Watchers campaign that says "Diets don't work." The message is that sensible eating is the answer to weight problems. We agree.

It doesn't help at all when you ask a doctor about your weight problem. The answer is likely to be, "You need to eat less and exercise more." They are still thinking in a linear manner; that is (calories ingested – calories burned = leftover calories that turn into fat). There's far more to weight gain than that, since we all burn calories differently, based on our inidividual body's metabolic efficiency.

Yes, you may be eating too much—or not. You may not be exercising enough—or not doing the right kind of exercise for your needs. Let's look at the underlying premise of the Vibrant Health Plan: if you're overweight, why? If you're eating too much, why? If you're not exercising enough, why not? The answer clearly lies in some systemic imbalance, and you probably have a good idea of which imbalance you're addressing by this time.

Weight is such an overwhelming concern for women that we've decided to give the problem its own chapter.

We believe that a healthy and balanced body will attain its appropriate weight—and stay there.

Being overweight is not a *disease* in itself, but it's an important sign of something being out of balance. We're here to help you figure out what that is and to address it through the earlier chapters. Think of this section as your jump start for approaching your weight issues and addressing body, mind, and spirit.

There are numerous causes of being overweight. Hormonal fluctuations (Chapter 11), thyroid malfunction (Chapter 12), chronic adrenal overload (Chapter 12), unbalanced blood sugar (Chapter 13), food allergies (Chapter 14), neurotransmitter imbalances that lead to uncontrolled food cravings (Chapter 10), and even bad genetics can cause susceptibility to weight gain that is difficult to reverse.

It's essential for you to understand this from the outset: these problems may have nothing to do with lack of discipline or slothful habits. They are very possibly systemic imbalances that can be corrected with the right supplements and the right diet.

In other words: *YOU ARE NOT TO BLAME! But you're responsible for taking the steps to solve the problem.*

Read these words several times. Integrate them into your psyche. Let them become part of your cellular structure. Write them on post-it notes, and stick them all over your house. Guilt is the relentless predator that sabotages the best eating intentions. Lose it from your mental vocabulary.

Add these words of encouragement: There *is* something you can do that doesn't involve relegating your life to rabbit food.

The imbalances that may be causing your weight gain and your inability to keep weight off are addressed in the appropriate chapters. This chapter is meant to give you a general overview of weight problems and your relationship to food and give you some solid tools for making changes that will really work.

Have you yo-yo dieted throughout your adult life? Have you shed weight, regained it, added a few pounds more, and then started the whole frustrating battle over again with the next fad diet? If this sounds like you, you most likely have systemic imbalances that can be corrected.

This isn't a diet book, but we've written this special chapter on weight precisely because it is such an overwhelming concern for the vast majority of women. We'll let you in on a few universal secrets here.

ALL DIETS WORK, AND NO DIETS WORK

All diets work, and no diets work. What do we mean by this? We mean that each of us is biologically unique. We've mentioned this before, and perhaps there is no other place where the concept of bio-individuality is as apparent as in the diet dilemma.

Even though we all love to share our stories of success and failure, what works for one woman may not work for anyone else.

Sure, there are some commonalities. The camaraderie offered by programs like Weight Watchers and Jenny Craig is a large part of their success. The loss of that fellowship is probably a large contributor to the rebound weight gain when successful dieters stop attending the weekly weigh-ins and meetings.

Everyone has a neighbor or a cousin who shed 50 pounds on the grapefruit diet or the cabbage soup diet.

We'll tell you that all of them are good—and all of them are bad.

We'll tell you something even more revolutionary: We don't believe in diets. Caution: Before you take this as permission to start the bacon double-cheeseburger/chocolate cake diet, we have to let you know we are firm believers in sensible eating.

We believe in eating lots of fruits and veggies, reasonable portions of good-quality meats and other proteins, plus high-quality complex carbohydrates like whole grain breads and pastas, the best quality vegetable and seed oils you can get, and indulgences within reason.

KATHLEEN'S STORY

Kathleen says she's always known that the first three letters of diet are *d-i-e*. She's struggled with her own weight problem since she reached perimenopause.

Here's her story:

When I had a partial hysterectomy due to fibroids and endometriosis at the age of 41 in 1989, we Boomers hadn't quite come into our own. Little was understood or discussed about menopause. It was "The Change" that our mothers whispered about in dire tones. No one talked about it. No one knew anything about it. Not even my doctor.

So I was blindsided when hot flashes from hell hit me shortly after the surgery. I didn't know what was happening, and I had no idea what to do about it. The lights came on about six months later when I had a meltdown in front of my mother and she announced in stentorian tones, "You're in menopause."

That wasn't possible, I whined to myself. I'm only 41! Along with hot flashes from hell came those "little" weight additions. I rationalized I was gaining only about five pounds a year. That's not much, is it? After, all, I *was* getting older. It didn't seem like much until I woke up one morning 10 years later and realized I had gained 50 pounds! Yikes.

I won't tell you I have all the answers, but I may have some handle on my own eating and craving patterns that can help some of you.

First, perimenopause wasn't my only problem.

As a journalist working in war zones at the time, I was seriously in the throes of toxic stress, even if no one had yet invented the term. I'd always had low blood pressure, and doctors had told me that was a good thing. Only when I began writing this book did I realize it means I probably have adrenal exhaustion, probably from a toxic stress overload!

My thyroid hormones were clearly out of whack, although two different doctors who measured my TSH levels declared my thyroid function was "normal." Dr. Cass reviewed my lab tests, took a clinical history, and prescribed desiccated (Armour) thyroid, 120 mg daily. The results were quite noticeable: I had more energy and could last all day without falling asleep at the computer or feeling that I needed a nap. I was my old self—and felt as good as I did 20 years ago!

Plus, in the midst of writing this book, she diagnosed me with candida! What a morass!

Now that I know what's going wrong, I'm able to address it. No, I'm not taking it all on at once. You know how to eat an elephant? One bite at a time. . . .

I've made some simple changes.

I love eating mini-meals. I eat about six times a day—each meal in the 300-calorie range. I try not to go more than three waking hours without eating something and that seems to balance my sugars and keep me satisfied.

I also started on thyroid pills, and, after a time, I went on natural hormone replacement.

The treadmill in my basement gets a three-mile workout every day, plus there are hikes and other excursions into my beloved Blue Ridge Mountains that are literally my backyard.

Do I obsessively count calories? No. Is it working? I won't tell you I've shed all 50 pounds, but it's starting to come off, a pound or two a week. That's where I want to be because I think it's more likely to stay off if it comes off slowly.

How do I feel? I feel better than I've felt in years. My energy is back, my bones are less achy, my mind is clearer and focused, and most important, I like myself again. I realize that this weight wasn't my fault but the product of a number of imbalances. Now that I know what's going on, I'm in charge, and it feels wonderful!

ABOUT THAT BACON DOUBLE-CHEESEBURGER AND CHOCOLATE CAKE

If you're walking the minefield of diet plans, you know how confusing it can be. Carbs are bad. No, carbs are good. Never eat margarine, but butter is bad, too. No, wait! Maybe some margarines are OK. Don't even think about eating a hamburger. No, hamburgers are great, but don't eat fruit or pasta. And on and on and on . . .

If you're confused, you're not alone. There is so much information available, and there are so many books and rigid diet plans that recent surveys show most of us are thoroughly confused about appropriate eating.

How do you know what's right? You don't. If you're exceptionally in tune with your own body, you may be able to tell what's good for you and what's not. Most of us aren't that in touch with our inner workings, so it's probably a good idea to think about some really general guidelines. Here are a few:

Portion Control

These days of triple-cheeseburgers and super-sized everything have left most of us uncertain about appropriate portion sizes. We've been encouraged to eat too much without even thinking about it and most likely have blunted our satiety receptors, the triggers in our brain that tell us when we're full.

IT'S ALL IN YOUR HANDS

- Three ounces of meat, poultry, or fish are about the size of a woman's palm or a deck of playing cards.

- One-half cup of cut fruit, vegetables, or pasta is about the size of a small fist.

- One cup of milk, yogurt, or chopped fresh greens is about the size of a small hand holding a tennis ball.

- An ounce of cheese is about the size of a thumb.

- A teaspoon of butter is about the size of a thumb tip.

A really helpful tip: if you're thinking about going back for seconds, wait a few minutes. Sip a little water and see if your desire for more food disappears. It takes 15 minutes for your stomach and brain to agree that you've had enough.

Fats Don't Make You Fat

Since the inception of the low-fat craze in the early {'}80s, Americans have become fatter and fatter and fatter because we're eating too much sugar and too many processed, nutritionally void foods. The best fats come from oils, seeds, and fish, and eating these regularly will definitely not cause weight gain. Omega-3 and omega-6 fatty acids are essential to optimal function of virtually every body system. They're especially important for good brain and cardiovascular function.

Animal fats are not all bad; however, we recommend avoiding highly processed animal fats like bacon, luncheon meats, hot dogs, and sausage because they're likely to be loaded with preservatives and additives. Another good reason to avoid high-fat animal products including meats and cheeses is that toxins are stored in fat, including animal fat. Of course, you'll want to avoid hydrogenated fats that remain solid at room temperature because they are harmful to cardiovascular health. That includes most margarines, Crisco and similar products, and baked goods made from these products. We believe that all highly processed foods, especially those laden with table sugar, are the primary contributors to overweight.

Mini-Meals Rock

Instead of eating three large meals a day, try eating five or six small meals spaced not more than three hours apart during your waking time. A recent Czechoslovakian study showed that people who ate five or more meals a day had half the chance of being overweight as those who ate only three meals. Plus they had a 60% reduced risk of high cholesterol and a 40% lower chance of having impaired blood sugars. The big difference comes from keeping your blood sugars stable and avoiding the fluctuations that cause cravings and overeating.

The key to success with the mini-meal plan is to take the number of calories you intend to eat during the day and divide it by the number of meals you intend to eat. For example, if your plan is to eat 1,800 calories during the day, divide it into six 300-calorie meals. This doesn't have to be precise. If you want to save some for a regular dinner with your family and then eat only an apple for your evening snack, that's fine. Your daily food diary might look like this:

- 7:00 a.m.—piece of whole grain toast with 1 tablespoon peanut butter and an apple

- 10:00 a.m.—piece of string cheese, three whole grain crackers, and handful of cherries

- 1:00 p.m.—half a turkey sandwich and a cup of vegetable soup or a salad (with small amount of dressing made from a healthy oil)

- 4:00 p.m.—small bran muffin and an orange

- 7:00 p.m.—poached salmon, $1/2$ cup of rice, broccoli, and a large salad with several vegetables (with small amount of dressing made from a healthy oil)

- 10:00 p.m.—two figs stuffed with cream cheese and almonds

Don't Skip Meals

Skipping meals is an invitation to overindulgence because you feel deprived, starved, and in search of a reward for your "good" behavior. Most weight-control experts agree that the biggest no-no is skipping breakfast. If you skip breakfast, your blood sugar crashes, and by lunchtime you're ready to eat everything in sight. It's all downhill from there. Whenever possible, eat within two hours after you wake up.

Kathleen's experience shows that eating a high-carb meal for breakfast, even a good one like a whole grain cereal, results in carb cravings all day long. For her, it's best to eat a high-protein breakfast and add carbs (like cereal) later in the day. A bowl of Kashi Go-Lean, fruit, and yogurt is her favorite lunch.

Try laying a good groundwork for your day with a breakfast of eggs, yogurt, or even a leftover chicken Caesar salad. No one ever said you have to eat breakfast food at breakfast time. Get creative and find out what works for you. Remember too that when you don't eat regularly, your metabolism slows down to accommodate the period of starvation. We still do have cave(wo)man bodies that respond to our environments. When you resume eating, you will burn calories at a slower rate, and you will have more trouble losing weight.

Here's something to consider: there's an adage that says eat breakfast like a king, lunch like a prince, and dinner like a pauper. It might work for you.

Take a Break

How often do you eat lunch at your desk? Or chow down in front of the TV? If you're eating alone, do you prop a book or a magazine in front of you? We women are famous multi-taskers, but there are times when it doesn't serve us well. Consider this: When you're focused on something other than eating, you'll eat more than if you are simply eating.

There was a time when families gathered for dinner to discuss the events of the day and share their triumphs and failures. Not many of us do that any more, and it is our loss, for many reasons.

Turn off the TV, put aside your book, ask a coworker to share lunch. When you eat, sit down at the table. Put your food on a plate (even if it's a snack food). Pay attention to what you're eating. Savor it.

You'll find you enjoy your food more, you'll stop eating sooner, and you'll grow closer to your family and friends.

Take time with your food. Chew each bite slowly. This allows your salivary enzymes to begin the digestive process, sending messages to your stomach to secrete hydrochloric acid and to the pancreas to release its enzymes and to prepare for the digestive process to continue. All of this engages the satiety center of your brain so you don't overeat.

Bringing consciousness to the eating and digestive process transforms the act of eating into a meditation. Another suggestion: before you begin eating, stop for a moment to give thanks for your food. Thank the land where your food grew. If the food is animal-based, thank the animal that gave away its life essence that your body might be nourished. Thank those who grew the food and those whose labor helped bring it to you. If you are comfortable with it, give thanks to whatever form of the Creator you honor. Ask that the food nourish your body, mind, and spirit.

Not only will this help you to be more conscious of the value of your food, but it will connect you to the larger web of life.

Attitude Adjustment

This is an easy one. You'll notice if you look back through this chapter that we've never used the words *weight loss.*

Remove them from your vocabulary! Thinking of losing something is a subconscious trigger that you are losing something important and that a part of you is going away. Reeducate yourself to think of shedding weight. After all, it's something you don't want, so why not shed? Think of healthy weight, weight normalizations, and best of all, weight control. After all, you're in charge!

Here's another helpful hint: Rearrange your mind to think of food as fuel. Many of us begin to think of food as a reward or as a crutch for emotional issues.

Another suggestion: Visualize yourself slim and healthy. If you have a picture of yourself at a time when you were comfortable with your weight, put it in a place where you can see it often to help your cellular memory readjust your weight to its normal level. If you don't have such a picture, draw one or stick your head on a magazine photo of someone else's gorgeous body.

FALLING OFF THE WAGON

So, you ate three pieces of pizza Saturday night. Or you couldn't stop once you dove into the Oreos. Falling off the wagon is the most common cause of weight-control failure. Have you ever thought, "Oh, well, I ate three pieces of pizza, so I might as well eat the whole thing"? Or, worse yet, "I'm a failure. I'll never lose weight. I'm destined to be a fat slob forever."

This kind of self-sabotage will only dig you deeper into your hole.

Recent research suggests that the reason for the failure of Atkins aficionados is not the weight-control plan itself, but the "falling off the wagon" stage when they go back to eating loads of carbs *on top of* all the meat, sausage, bacon, and cheese.

The problem with falling off the wagon is not a "moral" one; it is that if you are not balanced nutritionally, you could have a big fall. *If you are eating well and taking your supplements, these temptations are just not an issue.* This may be hard to believe for someone who hasn't tried this, but it's true.

Without micro-analyzing every bite you put in your mouth, if you have a slipup, look at it objectively and see what might be causing the cravings. If your slipup was for something sweet, look at Chapter 6. If you indulged in something salty and high in fat, consider that adrenal imbalance might be behind the craving and read Chapter 12.

One secret weapon for sugar-aholics, carb-aholics, and even alcoholics: you can cut your cravings enormously by balancing your brain chemistry. Simple interventions—such as emptying a capsule of glutamine powder under your tongue when the urge strikes—have stopped the hand that was about to seize a chunk of chocolate cake or a handful of potato chips or even a drink. For you chocolate lovers: Take your magnesium! Try it. Willpower is not needed: The craving just disappears!

YOUR CHOICE

Your choices are your own. You know your lifestyle, your body, and your level of determination better than anyone else.

We have some weight-control plans we like and others of which we are less fond. But, in the end, you'll be the one taking charge of your health and your weight, so choose a plan that you think will work for you.

Natural Supplements

Here is a list of supplements that help with both cravings and weight loss. In fact they all serve many roles in our complex and wonderful chemistry. Of course, begin with your multivitamin, fish oil and vitamin C.

Carb Blockers: White kidney bean extract manufactured under the name Phase 2 can safely block your body's absorption of starchy carbohydrates by 66%. Italian studies show that the carbohydrate blocker Phase 2 neutralizes as many as 2,250 carb calories in a day, so they pass right through your system without being converted to sugar and becoming fat. Sorry, but this does not include pure, refined sugar, which is absorbed almost immediately.
Cautions: May cause mild gas and bloating.
Doseage: Take 1,000–1,500 mg before each of your two meals highest in carbohydrates.

Chromium: Among other things, chromium increases the power of insulin to produce the brain chemical serotonin, which numerous studies have shown curbs appetite. About 90% of American adults are deficient in chromium, which keeps glucose levels under control, manages blood sugar over the long term, and fights insulin resistance. It also helps with weight control. It's sold as both chromium picolinate and chromium nicotinate.
Cautions: Safe at recommended doses. Do not exceed 1,200 mcg daily. High doses have been associated with kidney and liver damage. Do not exceed 200 mcg per day if you're pregnant or nursing.
Dosage: For dealing with blood sugar imbalances, take 500 mcg twice a day. For weight management, take up to 400 mcg a day for eight weeks.

Garcinia Cambogia: This East Indian fruit derivative works in several ways: it inhibits conversion of sugar into fat, curbs your appetite, aids in digestion, and reduces sweet cravings. It also appear to lower cholesterol and triglycerides.
Cautions: None.
Dosage: Take 500 mg three times a day, standardized to 50% hydroxycitric acid.

L-Glutamine: Glutamine curbs sugar cravings by as much as 50%. As the most common amino acid found in muscle tissues, glutamine improves both mental energy and relaxation, reduces addiction, stabilizes blood sugar, and promotes memory. Glutamine naturally elevates levels of growth hormone in your body, making your cells multiply faster, and slows aging. Additional amounts of growth hormone help mobilize fat from storage and make it available for energy.

Cautions: Do not use if you have kidney or liver disease.

Dosage: Take up to four 500 mg capsules daily with your regular supplements, or add glutamine powder to a protein drink (without sugar). Best taken about 30 minutes before a meal for fat management or at bedtime to enhance growth hormone production.

Gymnema Sylvestre: This well-researched Ayurvedic herb helps reduce both cravings for sweets, and sugar absorption in the intestine. It has been shown to lower glycosylated hemoglobin (Hb-A1C) in diabetics and to restore energy and well-being.

Cautions: If you're already on oral diabetic medications, you must monitor your glucose levels carefully.

Dosage: Take 100–200 mg daily.

L-Carnitine: A deficiency of the amino acid L-carnitine, which is contained in meat and dairy products, can be a major cause of weight gain. Vegetarians often need a boost of carnitine. It helps increase energy, burn fat, and support heart and liver health. Carnitine improves insulin sensitivity, protects against diabetic neuropathy, and helps keep blood fats (triglycerides) low and HDL or "good" cholesterol high. It also improves brain function and mental sharpness, and reduces stress.

Cautions: At higher doses, it can cause gastrointestinal problems. If this happens, lower the dosage and gradually build back up to your optimal level. Avoid taking L-carnitine after 3 p.m. because it may interfere with sleep. Some people report exceptionally vivid dreams, so adjust your dose accordingly.

Dosage: Take 500–4,000 mg daily (up to 2,000 mg twice daily), depending on your reason for using the supplement. For weight loss or if have seriously high triglycerides, go toward the higher end.

Essential Fatty Acids: EFAs (as Omega-3 fatty acids) release the hormone cholecystokinin from the stomach to the brain, telling you that you are full and keeping you feeling full for up to six hours after you eat.

Fish oil contains the essential fatty acids EPA and DHA, while flax oil contains only EPA.

Cautions: EPA and DHA help reduce blood clotting. High doses should not be taken if you are on blood-thinning medication.

Dosage: Take 1,000 mg once or twice a day as a fish oil supplement or eat 3 ounces of fatty fish three times a week. For weight management, look for a combination essential fatty acid that contains omega-3 and omega-6 oils. Always take with 400 IU of vitamin E daily as an antioxidant to prevent the oil's becoming rancid in your body.

Green Tea: Green tea boosts metabolism with its combination of caffeine and epigallocatechin gallate (ECGC) It stimulates the burning of brown or stored fat, and this continues for 24 hours after you take it. In addition, green tea boosts the immune system, protects against cancer and heart disease, normalizes blood sugars, and because of its theanine content, brings about a calm, focused feeling.

Cautions: Green tea still contains caffeine but does not seems to raise blood pressure and heart rate. However, use caution if you are sensitive to caffeine or other stimulants.

Dosage: Take 1–2 cups daily, or for greater effect, take capsules containing 50 mg of caffeine and 90 mg of ECGC per dose.

Tyrosine: This amino acid, also known as L-tyrosine, improves the burning of fats by boosting your metabolism, since it's a precursor to thyroid hormone. It also enhances mood and energy levels since it helps produces the stimulating neurotransmitters dopamine and norepinephrine, and the adrenal hormone epinephrine (adrenaline).

Cautions: Use caution if you have hypertension (high blood pressure). May cause mild gastrointestinal discomfort in some individuals.

Dosage: Take 500 mg twice daily. The therapeutic range is higher, and I have often successfully prescribed up to 3,000 mg a day in divided doses to depressed patients.

Milk Thistle (*Silybum Marianum*) or Silymarin: Milk thistle is a lipotropic (fat-burning) herb, useful for weight loss. It also has been shown to improve glucose intolerance, and to protect kidney cells from the toxic effects of glucose. A potent antioxidant, it speeds up detoxification and helps the liver regenerate after the process is complete.

Cautions: None.

Dosage: For glucose intolerance, take 200 mg of a standardized product daily. To deal with environmental toxins, take up to 650 mg daily. For weight management, take 30–60 mg three times a day.

You will find various combinations of these ingredients in the many supplement formulas on the market. Be sure they have enough of the ingredients to make a difference. The individual nutrients work together to boost each others' effects, so some ingredients may be at dosages slightly lower than we recommend.

One formula that I have found especially effective is Natural Chemistry's Weight Management Formula which I formulated, based on many of these ingredients. It is especially helpful when combined with Cellu-Detox, which aids detox through both the lymphatic system and the liver. (www.drcass.com)

WEIGHT AND HEALTH MAINTENANCE: WORK IN PROGRESS

Weight management, like good health, requires a multi-faceted approach. First, determine your particular weak spots, be it thyroid deficiency, gut dysbiosis or simply a poor diet, among others. Begin remedying that situation, while starting to deal with the whole picture: attitude, exercise, diet and supplements. Each aspect will reinforce the others, as you move toward creating your best self.

Please continue to review sections of this book as various questions or conditions arise. Redo the questionnaire periodically to monitor your progress. You may be surprised at how far you've come! Please also email me at www.drcass.com with questions, comments, and suggestions. Here's to your good health!

18

WHERE TO
LOOK FOR HELP

You now have many tools to help you achieve vibrant health, including books, newsletters and websites. You can subscribe to our free e-letters on www.drcass.com and www.kathleenbarnes.com, where you will find the latest health updates.

How to Find an Understanding Doctor

An ever-growing number of doctors in all specialties are coming to realize the role that nutrient deficiencies and toxicities can play in your health. If you are looking for one who shares this point of view, we have listed organizations of alternative physicians later in this chapter. If you are considering natural hormone therapy, be sure your doctor is familiar (and skilled) with its use.

You would need an M.D. (doctor of medicine) or D.O. (doctor of osteopathy) to write prescriptions for certain lab tests and for medications such as bioidentical hormones. There are laboratories that allow you to order tests through their physicians, with personnel available to help you interpret the tests. Besides medical doctors, these are some of the health care practitioners that you might consider consulting. Some of the more common alternative medicine practitioners may be covered by your medical insurance.

Osteopathic physicians (D.O.s) learn spinal-manipulation techniques and nutrition along with conventional medical training. However, many prefer to practice as conventional medical doctors, so ask before you make any assumptions. See www.osteopathic.org.

Naturopaths (N.D.s) study natural medicine in four-year accredited programs, which are making an enormous contribution to research and education in the field of natural medicine. Unfortunately, naturopaths are not yet licensed in all states. See www.naturopathic.org, or call (866) 538-2267.

There are non-licensed naturopaths from correspondence programs (not to be confused with the accredited ones). They can also be helpful with your nutritional needs.

Doctors of Oriental medicine (O.M.D.s) are licensed in all states to practice herbal medicine and acupuncture. Acupuncture can be an excellent way of regulating imbalances. See www.acupuncture.com.

Chiropractors (doctors of chiropractic, or D.C.s) can also be helpful—not simply in dealing with spines, bones, and muscles, either. Many are skilled in clinical nutrition as well as subtler forms of healing. See www.amerchiro.org.

Nutritionists are varied in their training and experience and should each be taken on their own skills, the recommendations of others, and their affiliation with medical practitioners to whom they refer patients when appropriate.

Herbalists, like nutritionists, vary in their training and skills. Their background is more grass roots, based in traditional folk medicine. The American Herbalists Guild is a well-respected organization whose membership is by invitation and peer review (www.americanherbalistsguild.com).

It is of greatest importance that you like and trust your health care professional. You should feel both free to ask questions and confident that you are being taken seriously. The relationship is a sacred one, based on the ancient tradition of priest-healer, and is the basis for your healing process. Trust your own intuition, both in terms of who you choose to work with and the direction in which they take you.

A good doctor will pay attention to your ideas and be willing to learn from you as well. This is a new model, a partnership in healing. Your doctor is the resource, the expert, in medical information and practice, and you are the expert in how you feel. The idea is to respect each other's roles in this relationship and to each do your part in your path to vibrant health.

PRACTITIONER ORGANIZATIONS

American Academy of Environmental Medicine
www.aaem.org
(800) 884-2236

American Association of Naturopathic Physicians
www.naturopathic.org
(866) 538-2267

American Association of Oriental Medicine
www.aaom.org
(888) 500-7999

American Chiropractic Association
www.amerchiro.org
(800) 986-4636

American College for Advancement in Medicine (ACAM)
www.acam.org
(800) 532-3688

American Herbalists Guild
www.americanherbalistsguild.com
(770) 751-6021

American Holistic Health Association
www.ahha.org
(714) 779-6152

For physician referrals, go to "Medical" section at ahha.org/ahhaprs.htm.

American Holistic Medical Association
www.holisticmedicine.org

American Osteopathic Association
www.osteopathic.org
(800) 621-1773

The Center for the Improvement of Human Functioning (founded by the late Hugh Riordan, M.D.)
3100 North Hillside Avenue
Wichita, KS 67219
www.brightspot.org
(316) 682-3100

International Society for Orthomolecular Medicine
www.orthomed.org
(416) 733-2117

The ISOM is an organization of doctors and osteopaths who practice ortho-molecular and preventive medicine in the United States, Canada, and abroad.

NAET (Nambudripad's Allergy Elimination Techniques)
www.naet.com

Find information, practitioners, and professional training courses on a natural treatment for allergies.

DIAGNOSTIC TESTING LABORATORIES

You can order diagnostic home test kits from these and other sources directly or through my website (www.drcass.com)

These are some of the specialized labs I use in my practice. You will need a doctor's prescription.

Doctor's Data
www.doctorsdata.com
(800) 323-2784

Metametrix
ww.metametrix.com
(800) 221-4640

**Genova Diagnostics Laboratory
(formerly known as Great Smokies
Diagnostic Labs)**
www.gdx.net
(800) 522-4762

COMPOUNDING PHARMACIES

Compounding pharmacies supply individualized prescription items such as natural hormones not generally carried by regular pharmacies. You can also contact them to find practitioners in your area. They will do mail order.

Apothecure Pharmacy in Dallas, TX
www.apothecure.com
(800) 969-6601

**Great Earth Compounding
Pharmacy**
www.greatearthpharmacy.com
(323) 650-0025

HealthWorld Online
http://healthy.net/professionals/
compound.asp
(800) 927-4227

**International Academy of
Compounding Pharmacists (IACP)**
www.iacprx.org
(800) 927-4227

**Pharmaca Integrative Pharmacy:
various locations**
www.pharmaca.com

**Women's International Pharmacy
in Madison, WI**
www.womensinternational.com
(800) 279-5708

CHOOSING SUPPLEMENTS

Be sure to use standardized herbs. Why? Herbs are made up of many ingredients that work together. In standardized herbs, one main ingredient is designated the "marker," usually the most active one. For example, by using an active substance in the herb as a marker, the manufacturer can ensure that each batch has a similar strength. This does not mean, however, that the other ingredients are excluded from the product. They are still needed for the full effect.

SUPPLEMENTS AND RELATED PRODUCTS

There are hundreds of safe and effective supplements on the market. Here is a partial selection of products and manufacturers that I have found to be high quality and effective. An updated and more in-depth list can be found on my website (www.drcass.com) and includes links to suppliers. Many of the supplements are also available in health food stores.

When you go shopping for supplements, you may wonder why their labels don't show much in the way of useful information, such as telling you what they should be used for. The reason for this seemingly deliberate lack of vital information is the FDA's Dietary Supplement Health and Education Act (DSHEA, 1994), which set new guidelines regarding the quality, labeling, packaging, and marketing of supplements.

DSHEA allows manufacturers to make "structure and function claims." This means that a label can explain how a vitamin or herb affects the structure or function of the body. However, it can make no therapeutic or prevention claims, such as "treats headaches" or "cures the common cold." A vitex agnus castus label (i.e., a supplement label) can say, "helps maintain healthy hormone levels," but it cannot say, "treats PMS," despite that being your reason for taking it.

For herbs, look for ones that are standardized, to ensure that they contain the (main active) marker ingredient, and in the required amount. You won't "lose" the rest of the plant—it's still included for full benefits from the plant's medicinal actions. For more details on how to shop for herbs, see my *User's Guide to Herbal Remedies* (Basic Health, 2004).

To be sure that the supplement you are buying contains what is on the label and is of high quality, buy from reputable sources, such as the ones listed in Chapter 18 or on drcass.com.

To check on a particular supplement or category, see www.ConsumerLab. com, an independent testing organization that provides regular reviews of commercially available products, lists of warnings and recalled products, and a free e-letter, too. Note: They are a for-profit organization and charge for their listings, so they are not totally without bias (consumerlab.com).

Products

Here are some supplements I consider highly effective.

CALM Natural Mind Formula is a unique blend of nutrients that work throughout the day to keep you calm, as well as an excellent after-work and bedtime relaxant. **Dosage:** 2 capsules 1–3 times daily as needed.

Nightly CALM formula is CALM plus valerian to help you fall and stay asleep. Dosage: 3 capsules at bedtime.

ENERGY Balance Formula is a blend of energizing nutrients including adaptogens to help you maintain energy throughout the day. All three formulas were developed by me and are available only through www.drcass.com.

Tango
www.puretango.com
(866) 77-TANGO

Special herbal formula developed in China from traditional "essence herbs" that are known to enhance libido and increase strength and duration of orgasm for both men and women. (You'll receive a 5% discount if you mention this book.)

Suppliers

Vital Choice Seafood
www.vitalchoice.com
(800) 608-4825
Carries canned and fresh frozen fish, guaranteed high in omega-3 oils and low in toxins.

Vitamin Research Products
www.vrp.com
(888) 401-0967
Full catalog of high-quality supplements. Sign up for complimentary prescriptions program (use PIN #215287 for discount).

INFORMATIONAL WEBSITES
WITH FREE E-NEWSLETTERS

Alternative Medicine
www.alternativemedicine.com

A comprehensive and up-to-date informational site, free e-newsletter, and monthly publication.

DoctorYourself.com
www.doctoryourself.com

This is Dr. Andrew Saul's excellent self-health site.

HealthWorld Online
www.healthy.net

Comprehensive information on complementary and alternative medicine, books, practitioners, and products, and a full line of lab tests and supplements.

Mercola.com
www.mercola.com

This is Dr. Joseph Mercola's comprehensive natural health website.

CANCER INFORMATION

Cancer Options
www.canceroption.com

Cancer Options has developed specific complementary therapies that assist in the prevention, recurrence, and remission of cancer and also help extend the lives of those who suffer from cancer.

CANHELP
www.canhelp.com
(360) 437-2291

The Moss Reports
www.cancerdecisions.com
(718) 636-4433

Created by Ralph Moss, Ph.D., for general as well as individualized reports on specific cancers.

NEWSLETTERS AND JOURNALS

Healthsmart Today: Impakt Health
www.impakt.com

$12 per year

The Nutrition Reporter Monthly
www.nutritionreporter.com

$26 per year. Newsletter that summarizes recent medical research on vitamins, minerals, and herbs.

Taste for Life Magazine
www.tasteforlife.com
(603) 924 7271

Free at health food stores. Dr. Cass is a member of the editorial advisory board.

Total Health Magazine
www.totalhealthmagazine.com
(888) 316-6051

$16.95 per year. Dr. Cass is medical editor.

Townsend Letter for Doctors and Patients
www.townsendletter.com
(360) 385-6021

$54 per year. Excellent journal providing scientific information on a wide variety of alternative medicine topics.

Women's Health Letter
www.soundpub.com
(800) 728-2288

$39 per year; free e-letter. Excellent monthly newsletter edited by Nan Fuchs, Ph.D., and published by Soundview Publications, P.O. Box 467939, Atlanta, GA, 31146.

RESOURCES

The following resources are divided into a chapter-by-chapter list of recommended reading as well as some supplement sources, laboratories, practitioners, newsletters, and useful websites.

Please visit my website, www.drcass.com, for updates and products.

Chapter 1: Beginning Your Journey to Better Health

Further Reading

Batmanghelidj, F., *Water: For Health, For Healing, For Life: You're Not Sick, You're Thirsty!* (Warner Books, 2003).

Cass, Hyla, Supplement your Prescription: What Your Doctor Doesn't Know About Nutrition (Basic Health, 2008).

Duke, James, *Dr. Duke's Essential Herbs* (Rodale, 1999).

Hoffman, Ronald, *How to Talk to Your Doctor* (Basic Health, 2006).

Hoffman, Ronald, *Intelligent Medicine* (Fireside, 1997).

Liponis, Mark, and Hyman, Mark, *Ultraprevention* (Scribner, 2003). By the co-medical directors of the famous Canyon Ranch Spa.

Chapter 3: Diagnostic Lab Tests

Further Reading

Heber, David, *The L.A. Shape Diet* (HarperCollins, 2004).

Simone, Charles B., *The Truth About Breast Health: Breast Cancer, Prescription for Healing* (Princeton Institute, 2002).

Johnson, Ben, M.D. and Barnes, Kathleen, *The Secret of Heath: Breast Wisdom* (Morgan James, 2008).

Websites

Nan Fuchs's Women's Health Letter: womenshealthletter.com.

breastthermography.com.

Chapter 5: Balance Your Diet

Further Reading

Appleton, Nancy, *Lick the Sugar Habit* (Avery, 1999).

Cass, Hyla, *User's Guide to Vitamin C.* (Basic Health, 2002).

Heber, David, *What Color Is Your Diet?* (Regan Books, 2002). Explains how a daily variety of fruits and vegetables can ward off disease and contribute to healthy living.

Lieberman, Shari, *The Real Vitamin and Mineral Book* (Avery Penguin Putnam, 2003).

Zimmerman, Marcia, *Eat Your Colors: Maximize Your Health by Eating the Right Foods for Your Body Type* (Holt, 2001). A consumer guide to discovering individual nutrition needs, based on food color and type, by the author of *The ADD Nutrition Solution* (Owl, 1999), another great resource.

Websites

For ginger and other pure concentrated herbal cooking extracts: www.primalessence. com.

For information on vitamins, minerals, and other supplements: vitamins: www. nutrition.org.

For nutrient content of specific foods: nal.usda.gov/fnic/foodcomp/search.

Chapter 6: Detoxify Your Body

Further Reading

Bennet, Peter, *7-Day Detox Miracle* (Prima Lifestyles, 2001).

Gittleman, Ann-Louise *The Fat Flush Plan* (McGraw-Hill, 2002).

Haas, Elson, *The Detox Diet: A How-To & When-To Guide for Cleansing the Body* (Celestial Arts, 1996).

Chapter 7: Exercise and Self-Care

Further Reading

Gittleman, Ann-Louise, *The Fat Flush Plan* (McGraw-Hill, 2002).

Seibel, Machelle, and Khalsa, Hari Kaur, *A Woman's Book of Yoga* (Avery, 2002).

Yoga

Kripalu Yoga Retreat: (800) 741-7353, www.kripalu.org.

White Lotus Yoga: (805) 964-1944, www.whitelotus.org. Offers books, tapes, teacher training, and retreats. Located in Santa Barbara, CA.

Meditation and transformation

BrainSync tapes and CDs with Kelly Howell: (800) 984-SYNC, www.brainsync.com.

Insight Meditation Society: (978) 355-4378, www.dharma.org.

Journey to Wild Divine: An enchanting program that uses biofeedback to teach breathing and meditation, and enhance relaxation www.wilddivine.com

Chapter 9: De-Stress Your Life

Further Reading

Cass, Hyla, and McNally, Terrence, *Kava: Nature's Answer to Stress, Anxiety, and Insomnia* (Prima, 1999).

Levine, Peter, *Waking the Tiger* (North Atlantic Books, 1997).

Sapolsky, Robert, *Why Zebras Don't Get Ulcers: An Updated Guide to Stress, Stress Related Diseases, and Coping* (W H Freeman & Co., 1998).

Recommended Products

CALM Natural Mind formula for reducing the stress response: www.drcass.com or (866) 778-2646.

Teeccino, a delicious herbal caffeine-free substitute that is prepared just like coffee and is available in health food stores: www.teeccino.com.

Chapter 10: Balancing Your Brain Chemistry

Further Reading

Amen, Daniel, *Change Your Brain, Change Your Life: The Breakthrough Program for Conquering Anxiety, Depression, Obsessiveness, Anger, and Impulsiveness* (Three Rivers Press, 1999).

Baker, Dan, *What Happy People Know: How the New Science of Happiness Can Change Your Life for the Better* (St. Martin's Griffin, 2004).

Brown, Richard, and Bottiglieri, Teodoro, *Stop Depression Now: SAM-e* (Berkley Books, 2000).

Cass, Hyla, *User's Guide to Ginkgo Biloba* (Basic Health, 2002).

Cass, Hyla, and Holford, Patrick, *Natural Highs: Diet Supplements and Mind-Body Techniques to Feel Good All the Time* (Avery, 2002).

Cohen, Jay, *Over Dose* (Tarcher/Putnam, 2001).

Gant, Charles, *End Your Addiction Now: The Proven Nutritional Supplement Program That Can Set You Free* (Warner Books, 2002).

Glenmullen, Joseph, *Prozac Backlash* (Touchstone Books, 2001). Describes the adverse effects of Prozac and other SSRI antidepressants.

Holford, Patrick, *Optimum Nutrition for the Mind* (Basic Health, 2004) (New edition: Piatkus Press, London 2007).

Larson, Joan Matthews, *End Depression Naturally* (Random House, 2000). Excellent resource for treating depression with supplements.

Larson, Joan Matthews, *Seven Weeks to Sobriety: The Proven Program to Fight Alcoholism Through Nutrition* (Ballantine Books, 1997).

Sahelian, Ray, *Mind Boosters* (St. Martin's Griffin, 2000).

Stone, Hal, and Sidra Stone, *Embracing Our Selves: The Voice Dialogue Manual* (Nataraj, 1993). The Stones have many other excellent books on the Voice Dialogue process (including *Partnering: A New Kind of Relationship* (New World Library, 2000).

Websites

alternativementalhealth.com.

Daniel Amen: www.amenclinic.com, www.brainplace.com.

Voice Dialogue process: www.delos-inc.com.

Chapter 11: Sex Hormones: From PMS to Menopause

Further Reading

Ahlgrimm, Marla, and Kells, John, *The HRT Solution* (Avery, 2003).

Barnes, Kathleen, *User's Guide to Natural Hormone Replacement* (Basic Health, 2006).

Berkson, D. Lindsey, *Hormone Deception* (McGraw-Hill/Contemporary Books, 2001).

Berkson, D. Lindsey, *Natural Answers for Women's Health Questions* (Fireside Books, 2002).

Kahmi, Ellen, *Cycles of Life* (M. Evans, 2001).

Laux, Marcus, and Conrad, Christine, *Natural Woman, Natural Menopause* (HarperCollins, 1997).

Lieberman, Shari, *Get Off the Menopause Roller Coaster* (Avery, 2000).

Northrup, Christiane, *The Wisdom of Menopause* (Bantam, 2003).

Northrup, Christiane, *Women's Bodies, Women's Wisdom* (Bantam, 2002).

Reiss, Uzzi, *Natural Hormone Balance for Women* (Atria, 2002).

Riess, Uzzi, *The Natural Superwoman* (Avery 2008).

Somers, Suzanne, *The Sexy Years 2002* (Random House, 2004).

Somers, Suzanne, *Ageless: The Naked Truth About Bioidentical Hormones* (Crown Books, 2006).

Stengler, Angela, and Stengler, Mark, *Your Menopause, Your Menotype* (Avery, 2003).

Watson, Cynthia, *User's Guide to Easing Menopause Symptoms Naturally* (Basic Health, 2003).

Chapter 12: Thyroid and Adrenals: Your Energy Glands

Further Reading

Barnes, Kathleen, *User's Guide to Thyroid Disorders* (Basic Health, 2006).Hanley, Jesse Lynn, *Tired of Being Tired* (Penguin Putnam, 2000).

Jeffries, Williams, *Safe Uses of Cortisol* (Charles C. Thomas, 1996).

Schwarzbein, Diane, *The Schwarzbein Principle II: The "Transition"—A Regeneration Program to Prevent and Reverse Accelerated Aging* (Health Communications, 2002). Includes information on the relationship between adrenal stress and insulin resistance.

Shames, Richard, and Shames, Karilee, *Thyroid Power* (Quill, 2002).

Shomon, Mary, *Living Well with Chronic Fatigue Syndrome and Fibromyalgia: What Your Doctor Doesn't Tell You . . . That You Need to Know* (HarperResource, 2004).

Shomon, Mary, *Living Well with Hypothyroidism* (Quill, 2000).

Siegal, Sanford, and Gaby, Alan. *Is Your Thyroid Making You Fat?* (Warner Books, 2001).

Talbott, Shawn, *The Cortisol Connection* (Hunter House, 2002).

Teitelbaum, Jacob, *From Fatigued to Fantastic* (revised edition) (Avery, 2007).

Home Lab Testing

See www.drcass.com for details.

Websites

Broda Barnes Foundation (information and physician referrals): www.brodabarnes. org. Also call (203) 261-2101.

www.cfsfibromyalgia.com.

Dr. Jacob Teitelbaum: www.endfatigue.com.

Mary Shomon: www.thyroid-info.com, www.thyroid.about.com, www.adrenal fatigue. org.

Chapter 13: Metabolic Syndrome X and Blood Sugar Imbalances

Further Reading

Challem, Jack, Burton Berkson, and Melissa Diane Smith, *Syndrome X* (Wiley, 2000).

Challem, Jack, *Stop Prediabetes Now: The Ultimate Plan to Lose Weight and Prevent Diabetes* (Wiley, 2007).

Chandalia J., A. Garg, D. Lutjohann, et al. "Beneficial Effects of High Dietary Fiber Intake in Patients with Type 2 Diabetes Mellitus." *New England Journal of Medicine.* 342 (19): 1440–41 (May 2000).

Reaven, Gerald, *Syndrome X* (Simon and Schuster, 2000).

Chapter 15: Environmental Toxin Imbalances

Further Reading

Berkson, D. Lindsey, *Hormone Deception: How Everyday Foods and Products Are Disrupting Your Hormones—and How to Protect Yourself and Your Family.* (Reprint, McGraw-Hill/Contemporary Books, 2001).

Carson, Rachel, *The Silent Spring,*40th-anniversary ed. (Houghton Mifflin, 2002).

Colborn, Theo. *Our Stolen Future: Are We Threatening Our Fertility, Intelligence, and Survival?—A Scientific Detective Story* (Plume, 1997).

Davis, Devra, *When Smoke Ran Like Water: Tales of Environmental Deception and the Battle Against Pollution* (Basic Books, 2003).

Davis, Devra, *The Secret History of the War on Cancer* (Basic Books, 2007).

Fuchs, Nan, *Modified Citrus Pectin (MCP): A Super Nutraceutical* (Basic Health, 2004). Supports the removal of a variety of toxins from the body.

Gittleman, Ann-Louise, *The Living Beauty Detox Program* (HarperCollins, 2000).

Rogers, Sherry, *Detoxify or Die* (Prestige Publishers, 2002).

Websites

Agency for Toxic Substances and Disease Registry: www.atsdr.cdc.gov.

Product information: www.econugenics.com.

Chapter 16: Musculoskeletal Pain: Headaches, Arthritis, and Osteoporosis

Further Reading

Barnes, Kathleen, *Arthritis and Joint Health* (Woodland, 2005).

Bic, Zuzanna, and Bic, L. Francis, *No More Headaches No More Migraines* (Avery, 1999).

Germano, Carl, and Cabot, William, *Nature's Pain Killers: Proven New Alternative and Nutritional Therapies for Chronic Pain Relief* (Kensington, 1999).

Germano, Carl, and Cabot, William, *The Osteoporosis Solution* (Kensington, 1999).

Jacob, Stanley, Lawrence, Ronald and Zucker, Martin, *The Miracle of MSM* (Berkley Books, 1999).

Newmark, Thomas, and Schulick, Paul, *Beyond Aspirin* (Hohm Press, 2000).

Sarno, John, *Healing Back Pain: The Mind-Body Prescription* (Warner, 1991).

Websites

National Arthritis Foundation: www.arthritis.org.

National Headache Foundation: www.headaches.org.

National Osteoporosis Foundation: www.nof.org.

Chapter 17: Managing Your Weight

Further Reading

Cherniske, Stephen, *The Metabolic Plan* (Ballantine Books, 2003).

Fuchs, Nan, *Overcoming the Legacy of Overeating: How to Change Your Negative Eating Patterns* (McGraw-Hill, 1999).

Gittleman, Ann-Louise, *The Fat Flush Plan* (McGraw-Hill, 2002).

Gittleman, Ann-Louise, *The Fat Flush Cookbook.* (McGraw-Hill, 2003).

Gittleman, Ann-Louise, *The Fat Flush Fitness Plan* (McGraw-Hill, 2004).

Hass, Elson, and Stauth, Cameron, *The False Fat Diet* (Ballantine, 2001).

Heber, David, *The L.A. Shape Diet: The 14-Day Total Weight Loss Plan* (Regan Books, 2004).

Hyman, Mark, *Ultrametabolism: The Simple Plan for Automatic Weight Loss* (Atria, 2008).

Lieberman, Shari, *Dare to Lose: Four Simple Steps to Achieve a Better Body* (Avery-Penguin Putnam, 2003). A combined strategy of sensible eating, exercise, relaxation techniques, and the use of over-the-counter weight-loss supplements.

Peeke, Pamela, *Fight Fat After Forty* (Viking, 2000).

Websites

A list of foods with their fiber content, as well as articles and recipes: www.fatfree kitchen.com/fiberlist.

Chapter 18: Where to Look for Help

Cass, Hyla, *User's Guide to Herbal Remedies* (Basic Health, 2004).

INDEX

D

ABOUT THE
AUTHORS

Hyla Cass, M.D., has integrated functional medicine with psychiatry in her clinical practice of over twenty years, and is a noted public speaker, consultant, and educator on integrative medicine and psychiatry, women's health, and natural treatments for anxiety disorders, depression and addiction. She is also a frequent commentator in newspapers, magazines, radio, and television, and contributor to numerous books and journals. She has appeared on such TV shows as *The View, MSNBC,* and *PBS;* radio shows include National Public Radio and Mehmet Oz's Oprah & Friends Radio.

Dr. Cass graduated from the University of Toronto School of Medicine, interned at Los Angeles County-USC Medical Center, and completed a psychiatric residency at Cedars-Sinai Medical Center. Dr. Cass is the author of 10 books, including *Natural Highs: Supplements, Nutrition and Mind-Body Techniques, 8 Weeks to Vibrant Health,* and *Supplement Your Prescription: What Your Doctor Doesn't Know About Nutrition.* For more information see her website www.drcass.com.

Kathleen Barnes has pursued her passion for natural health for more than thirty years, as a teacher of yoga and other spiritual practices and, in recent years, as a magazine writer and author and editor of a round dozen books on natural health and sustainable living. She is also editor of her own newsletter and website, Living, Naturally. You can find it and more information at www. kathleenbarnes.com.

Kathleen graduated from Purdue University with a degree in journalism and spent many years as a newspaper reporter before she became a foreign correspondent, covering Europe, Asia and Africa for ABC News, CNN, Canadian Television and a host of international publications. She wrote a natural health column for *Woman's World* magazine for six years before deciding to devote her career to writing books.

Among her books are *The Secret of Health: Breast Wisdom* written with Dr. Ben Johnson, *Basic Health User's Guide to Thyroid Disorders* and *Basic Health User's Guide to Natural Hormone Replacement.*

A PERSONAL NOTE FROM DR. CASS

I hope this book has empowered you on your path to a happier, healthier life. For continuous updates, please visit my website at www.drcass.com, where you will find the following:

Free E- newsletter: Sign up for the latest natural health news.

FAQs: Answers to frequently asked health questions

Resources and links: For related books, articles, and services

Products: Sources of high quality supplements.

Events calendar: Listing of my radio and TV interviews, lectures, and workshops.

Reader Feedback: I would enjoy hearing from you. Let me know how this book has affected your life, as well as what information you would like to see in future books and articles. You can e-mail me at dr@drcass.com.

Consultations: I have a private practice in the Los Angeles area. For further information, see my website.

Wishing you a lifetime of good health!

Hyla Cass, MD